Manual of Fetal Echocardiography

If you can trust yourself when all men doubt you
But make allowance for their doubting too.

If by Rudyard Kipling

This book is dedicated to all those people throughout my life who have inspired me by telling me that my proposed next step was impossible; also to Chris, Nick and Kim, who make it all worthwile.

Manual of Fetal Echocardiography

Lindsey D. Allan, MD, MRCP

Senior Lecturer in Perinatal Cardiology and Honorary Consultant, Guy's Hospital, London

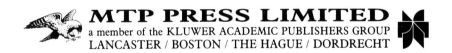

MTP PRESS LIMITED
a member of the KLUWER ACADEMIC PUBLISHERS GROUP
LANCASTER / BOSTON / THE HAGUE / DORDRECHT

Published in the UK and Europe by
MTP Press Limited
Falcon House
Lancaster, England

British Library Cataloguing in Publication Data

Allan, Lindsey D.
  Manual of fetal echocardiography.
  1. Fetal heart rate monitoring
  2. Ultrasonic cardiography
  I. Title
  618.3'26107543   RG628.3.H42

ISBN 0–85200–988–7

Published in the USA by
MTP Press
A division of Kluwer Academic Publishers
101 Philip Drive
Norwell, MA 02061, USA

Library of Congress Cataloging in Publication Data

Allan, Lindsey D. (Lindsey Dorothy)
  Manual of fetal echocardiography.

  Bibliography: p.
  Includes index.
  1. Fetal heart—Abnormalities—Diagnosis. 2. Fetal
heart—Anatomy. 3. Ultrasonic cardiography. 4. Prenatal
diagnosis. I. Title. [DNLM: 1. Echocardiography.
2. Fetal Heart—abnormalities. 3. Fetal Heart—anatomy
& histology. 4. Heart Defects, Congenital—diagnosis.
5. Prenatal Diagnosis. WQ 210.5 A417m]
RG628.3.H42A45 1986   618.3'26107543   86–21300
ISBN 0–85200–988–7

Typeset and printed by Butler & Tanner Limited, Frome and London

Contents

Abbreviations

These abbreviations are used throughout the illustrations.

AAo	ascending aorta
ACW	anterior chest wall
Ao	aorta
as	atrial septum
asd	atrial septal defect
ca	common atrium
CPV	common pulmonary vein
DA	ductus arteriosus
DAo	descending aorta
fo	foramen ovale
IVC	inferior vena cava
IVS	interventricular septum
la	left atrium
laa	left atrial appendage
LCCA	left common carotid artery
lpa	left pulmonary artery
LV	left ventricle
MPA	main pulmonary artery
Mv	mitral valve
Mv att.	mitral valve attachment
PA	pulmonary artery
pe	pericardial effusion
pl.eff or plE	pleural effusion
pv	pulmonary valve
ra	right atrium
rpa	right pulmonary artery

rrv	rudimentary right ventricle
RV	right ventricle
S	spine
sa	subclavian artery
st	stomach
SVC	superior vena cava
t	trachea
Tv	tricuspid valve
Umb cord	umbilical cord
UV	umbilical vein

Acknowledgements

I would like to acknowledge Professor Michael Tynan and Dr Michael Joseph for their moral support, as well as financial, enabling this work to start and continue. Professor Tynan is particularly thanked for constructive criticism and friendship over many years. I would like to thank Professor Robert Anderson for the anatomical illustrations in this book, for many specimen dissections in the last few years and much encouragement. I would like to express my gratitude to The British Heart Foundation for their generous support of the work of the department. Their funding has not only provided staff but also high quality scanning equipment allowing us the opportunity to maximize our expertise and accuracy. I would like to thank Dr Diane Crawford and Mrs Sunder Chita for performing the work of the department to such a high standard, Dr Crawford having been a reliable friend and colleague for several years. I would like to thank Mrs Norah Ford, my secretary, for uncomplaining service over the years, for the retyping of numerous manuscripts, despite an ever-increasing clinical load.

Introduction

The aim of this book is to provide a photographic instruction manual and practical guide based on six years' learning experience[1-20]. It is hoped that it will be kept at hand in the scanning room for constant reference.

At first sight, the anatomy of the heart appears complicated to the non-cardiologist involved in fetal scanning, and in the first instance the cardiologist finds reversing and inverting cardiac images difficult in the fetal study. However, once some basic keys to orientation and interpretation are learnt, the fetal heart can be readily and completely examined by both groups. A thorough three-dimensional understanding of the anatomy of the thorax and the relations of the heart and great vessels is essential for fetal echocardiography, but this is less daunting than it first appears.

It should be remembered when approaching the fetal echocardiogram that no additional information is already available to help with diagnosis and no further information about the heart is going to be available before birth. There are no clinical signs, electrocardiogram, chest X-ray or catheterization data to assist in diagnosis. The patient is dependent on the operator's ability to interpret the echocardiogram alone. Important decisions on the management or outcome of the pregnancy will depend on this interpretation. We have therefore tried to illustrate fully the method of diagnosing structural normality, the accurate prediction of which is as important as that of structural abnormality. We have had a unique opportunity to document a nearly complete range of structural heart disease prenatally and feel that the illustrations of these examples should be of assistance to the obstetric ultrasonographer or experienced paediatric echocardiographer alike. A cross-section of videotapes acquired in routine patients has been used to illustrate normal fetal heart scanning such that a representative sample of image quality is presented. The moving image is of course much easier to understand and interpret than the still photographs. Freezing one frame loses all the information supplied by surrounding frames. The image quality achieved in the abnormal cases is not always perfect and the pictures obtained are the best available in the circumstances. Frequently these circumstances are not ideal, e.g. late gestation, hydramnios etc., such that a wide variation in image quality is achieved in cases of anomaly. We have also tried to draw attention to potential sources of error which we have encountered and to our current estimation of the confidence limits of the technique with today's technology and experience.

CHAPTER 1

Normal fetal cardiac anatomy – cross-sectional echocardiography

The quality of cross-sectional images of the fetal heart achieved will depend on several factors:

(1) *The quality and type of equipment.* We have always used a sector scanner in fetal cardiac imaging. The small, easily held and manipulated probe can allow unhindered angulation around the maternal abdomen, an important facility for maximum evaluation. For the first five years we used an ATL mark III sector scanner. Since early 1985 we have used a Hewlett–Packard 77020A(HP). This gives us the additional facility of Doppler evaluation. The 5 mHz transducer is nearly always suitable, with medium focus on the HP. This gives resolution of 1–2 mm depending on the orientation of the beam to the scanned structure, axial being better than lateral resolution. Rarely the 3 mHz transducer is necessary in late pregnancy. The fetal heart in normal circumstances lies 1–10 cm from the transducer, usually 5–7 cm.

There is no objection to the use of linear array scanners, however. Many obstetric ultrasonographers, particularly when used to this type of equipment, can produce comparable images to those achieved by sector scanners. Occasionally, in our hands, we find pelvic angulation can be hampered by the size of a linear array transducer and this can be a disadvantage. The image quality produced by small, often portable, inexpensive recently developed equipment can be extremely good. If image quality alone is considered there can sometimes be little difference between equipments differing by £20000–40000 in price. M-mode and Doppler facility is important for specialist cardiological evaluation but is not necessary for basic scanning and the initial detection of a wide range of abnormalities. Thus, in the majority of patients nowadays, fetal cardiac analysis is within the scope of the ultrasound equipment available in most obstetric departments.

(2) *The gestational age.* The structure of the heart can be visualized from as early as 10 weeks gestation up to term. Figure 1.1 shows the arterial relations in a fetus of 10 weeks using computer assisted sonography with a zoom facility. With less powerful equipment four chambers of the heart can become identifiable by 14 weeks gestation. However, the position of the fetus lying anteroposteriorly in the uterus is often unfavourable at this time. For most practical circumstances, the most useful images are achieved by 18 weeks gestation. Imaging becomes more difficult towards term partly because of rib shadowing but also because of an often fixed fetal position with the anterior chest away from the transducer. In this situation, the greater distance that the beam needs to penetrate can limit image quality.

(3) *Maternal obesity and abdominal scarring.* Maternal obesity limiting image quality for all aspects of obstetric scanning is not an uncommon problem. It is unusual for it to completely preclude at least limited cardiac evaluation in the midtrimester. It is my impression that marked abdominal striae affect the quality of obstetric images adversely. But this will rarely prevent diagnostic cardiac analysis.

(4) *Oligohydramnios or polyhydramnios.* Both too much and too little amniotic fluid will affect the quality of the cardiac scan. All the fetal parts are difficult to see in oligohydramnios when the favourable effect of a fluid-filled sac for optimum transmission of ultrasound is lost. Polyhydramnios can make cardiac scanning difficult as the fetal thorax is often displaced a long distance, up to 20 cm, away from the transducer. This is not a problem if one is fortunate enough to have a zoom facility on the ultrasound scanner.

(5) *The fetal position.* This has an important influence on the adequacy of cardiac evaluation. There is never any need for filling the bladder even in early scanning as the heart will always be seen in the middle of the fetus whether the head or bottom is in the pelvis. Once methods of orientation are learnt it is immaterial whether the fetus lies head down, breech or transverse. The relative position of the spine to the transducer is, however, of great importance. The fetal heart will appear different, even when seen in the same section, with different positions of the spine. Also the spinal position can limit access to all the longitudinal sections of the fetal heart which can be seen. Often

moving around the abdomen and cutting in at an angle can overcome positional abnormalities.

In the midtrimester normal fetus, fetal movement will often change from an unfavourable to a favourable position during the scanning time or vice versa. Fetal truncal movement is usually of great advantage to the cardiac scanner, although images have to be recognized and structures identified quickly as they pass into and out of view. Lack of truncal movement in late pregnancy can restrict evaluation. Also a sick fetus will have diminished movement, increasing the difficulty of a study in this situation if the initial position is unfavourable.

(6)   *Extracardiac anomalies.* Distortion of the cardiac position by extracardiac anomalies can create difficulties in the interpretation of cardiac anatomy. Pleural effusions, absent lung on one side, diaphragmatic hernia and even exomphalos are all examples of conditions which may hamper complete cardiac evaluation. Not only are the venous and arterial connections distorted by such anomalies but the four-chamber view can be displaced from its normal intrathoracic position.

CROSS-SECTIONAL IMAGING

Fetal echocardiography cannot be directly compared to the postnatal study for several reasons. First, the fetal heart lies in a different orientation in the fetal thorax. The apex is displaced upwards into a more horizontal position by the large fetal liver (Figure 1.2). Also, the right ventricle is equal in size to the left ventricle and lies directly anterior to it instead of inferior to it as in postnatal life. The normal widely patent foramen ovale and ductus arteriosus are readily seen in prenatal life. The most important difference, however, is due to the fact that the lung fields are unaerated and fluid-filled in prenatal life. The unobstructed access to visualization of the fetal heart produces unusual images of the heart in projections unobtainable postnatally. This can lead to misinterpretation for the inexperienced, but usually the multiplicity of projections is helpful in diagnosis.

The easiest view to recognize and obtain is the four-chamber view of the heart. Because of the position of the heart referred to above, this view is achieved in a straight cut across the fetal thorax at the base of the sternum (Figure 1.3a). This section lies between the view of the abdomen necessary for measuring abdominal circumference and the view of the head necessary for measuring the biparietal diameter.

Therefore the obstetric ultrasonographer can readily achieve the four-chamber view of the heart by moving straight up or straight down from more familiar images. The thorax appears as a circular structure with the spine at any point on the circumference of this circle. The spine has the characteristic appearance of the bony vertebral body with the central circular canal (Figure 1.3b). To ensure that the section is not oblique at least one complete rib should be seen. Once the spine has been identified the sternum can be located lying directly opposite the spine in the centre of the anterior chest wall. The right ventricle lies underneath the sternum. The descending aorta lying anterior to the spine, seen as a circle in cross-section, is the next structure to be sought. It lies between the spine and left atrium. Once the right ventricle and left atrium are recognized the other intracardiac chambers can be easily identified. This method of orientation is illustrated in Figure 1.4.

The appearance of the four-chamber view will vary according to the fetal position, but no matter what the fetal position, the method of orientation starting from the spine should always be the same as that presented in Figure 1.4. The differing appearance of the four-chamber view is due to the different possible orientations of the ultrasound beam to the plane of the ventricular septum. Figure 1.5 illustrates the main possible approaches of the ultrasound beam to the fetal thorax. There are basically six possible orientations to the four-chamber view. In positions 1 and 3 (Figure 1.5) the ultrasound beam will be parallel to the ventricular septum. Position 1 will look identical to position 3, except for being inverted and less clear, the heart being further away from the ultrasound beam in position 1 than it is in position 3. Figures 1.6 and 1.7 are examples of the four-chamber view in positions 1 and 3 respectively.

The thickness of the ventricular walls is not clearly defined in these views because of physical limitations in lateral resolution. However, the crux of the heart is best seen in these projections illustrating the normal 'offset' appearance. This can be more clearly seen in the four-chamber view in Figure 1.8. This is due to the normal differential insertion of the two atrioventricular valves, the septal leaflet of the tricuspid valve being inserted slightly more apically than the mitral. The atrial septum, atrioventricular valves and ventricular septum can be seen to meet at the crux of the heart. Figure 1.8 also illustrates an important normal point to note in the four-chamber view – the heart occupies approximately one third of the fetal thorax. The coarser trabeculation and moderator band of the right ventricle can often be appreciated in this projection (Figure 1.7). In these views the foramen ovale often appears large. This is because of dropout in the atrial septum distal to the foramen where the resolution of the ultrasound beam is not sufficient to define the very thin septum when the beam is parallel to it. Similarly dropout or 'fading' of the ventricular septum is often noted just below the atrioventricular valves in these projections (Figures 1.6, 1.7 and 1.8). This is again because of the limited resolution capacity of the ultrasound equipment to define this thin part of the ventricular septum when the beam is parallel to it. Opening of the septal and lateral cusps of both atrioventricular valves are most clearly seen in these projections (Figure 1.9).

In positions 2 and 4 (Figure 1.5) the ultrasound beam will be perpendicular to the ventricular walls and septum. Because axial resolution is better than lateral resolution, wall and septal thickness in this projection will be more clearly defined. The margins of the foramen ovale can often be precisely defined. The flap valve can be seen flickering within the body of the left atrium. This is a prominent structure in fetal life. The atrioventricular valves to their respective chordal attachments can often be clearly identified. These features are shown in Figures 1.10 and 1.11, corresponding to positions 2 and 4 respectively. Figures 1.10 and 1.11 can be seen to be identical but inverted. As the heart in each case is a similar distance from the transducer, image quality will be similar in each position.

In position 5 (Figure 1.5) the appearance of the four-chamber view will be somewhere between the appearances of positions 2 and 4 and readily interpretable. If the fetal thorax is approached from position 6, the resultant image will depend on the gestational age. In early pregnancy (<24 weeks or so) the image achieved will be identical to that seen in position 5 but inverted. It will be readily intelligible. However, in later pregnancy the spine will shadow the heart and the operator has to move around the maternal abdomen to approach from positions 1 or 2. Figure 1.12 shows the spine close to the transducer completely obstructing the cardiac image. Moving towards position 1 allows the four-chamber view to be seen still partly shadowed. If the usual method of orientation is used the cardiac structures can be identified despite the shadow (Figure 1.13). Note that Figures 1.6 and 1.13 are four-chamber views in position 1, but lateral inversions of each other. The operator must familiarize himself not only with anterior–superior inversion, but also lateral inversion. However, if the same sequence is followed, using the spine for orientation each time, each intracardiac chamber can be accurately mentally labelled.

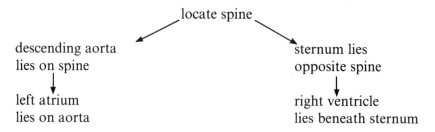

Whatever the fetal position the following points must be noted in the four-chamber view:

(1) The heart fills approximately 1/3 of the fetal thorax.
(2) The right and left atrial chambers are similar in size.
(3) The right ventricular cavity is approximately equal to the left ventricular cavity in size across the inlet of the ventricles (Figure 1.14).
(4) The posterior walls of right and left ventricles and inter-ventricular septum are approximately equal in thickness.
(5) The atrioventricular valves open with each cardiac cycle.
(6) The atrial and ventricular septa and atrioventricular valves meet together at the crux of the heart in an offset cross.
(7) The normal atrial defect can be seen.
(8) The ventricular septum appears intact.

If the heart is normal, all these points can be noted in every pregnancy from 16 weeks gestation to term. Occasionally because of spine or limb shadowing the transducer has to be moved from side to side to examine each of the four chambers separately. Instead of being able to note all the important points in one single slice, the points need to be put together from several angles. For example, in Figure 1.13 the crux of the heart and two atria can be seen. To compare ventricular size the spinal shadow would need to be swung to the right of the image.

Another normal feature which can be noted in the four-chamber view is the pulmonary venous connection. The pulmonary veins can be readily seen in prenatal life, clearly outlined passing into lung substance often as far as first generation branches. Pulmonary veins are illustrated in Figure 1.15. Contrary to estimates in the fetal lamb[21], pulmonary veins do appear to carry a significant volume of blood and they are of the same proportionate size relative to the other cardiac structures as in postnatal life.

Once the four-chamber view has been recognized and understood, the operator can proceed to look first at left and then at right heart connections. Whatever the orientation of the four-chamber view cranial angulation of the transducer produces 'five chambers' or a four-chamber aortic root view. This sequence is illustrated in Figures 1.16a and 1.16b. Additionally, twisting the transducer in this plane will open out the aorta so that the left ventricle is seen in long axis projection similar to that seen postnatally. In this view the left heart connections can all be recognized (Figure 1.17b). The transducer orientation to produce this view is seen in Figure 1.17a. One pulmonary vein can be seen entering the left atrium, the mitral valve connects to left ventricle, the left ventricle to a great artery which should be the aorta. However, this cannot be labelled the aorta until its connection to the arch and its head and neck vessels have been identified. This can be done, however, in a continuous sweep. The sequence is displayed in Figures 1.17b, 1.18 and 1.19b). Continuity between the ventricular septum and anterior wall of aorta and the anterior leaflet of the mitral valve and posterior wall of aorta are additional important normal features to note in the long axis of the left ventricle. The complete arch with three head and neck vessels are seen in Figure 1.19b. The transducer orientation for this plane is seen in Figure 1.19a. The right pulmonary artery can be seen in the hook of the arch. The arch must be seen as a 'tight' hook tucking into the centre of the chest quite a distance from the anterior chest wall. This will distinguish the arch from the ductal connection which is seen in Figure 1.20b. The transducer orientation required for this section is seen in Figure. 1.20a. The main pulmonary artery communication with the duct has no head and neck vessels arising from it, and arises from the right ventricle close to the anterior chest wall. The right heart connections are seen in this projection. The inferior vena cava is seen entering the right atrium through the diaphragm. The right atrium communicates via the tricuspid valve with the right ventricle. The right ventricle and infundibulum 'wraps' around the aorta, seen in cross-section in the centre of this scan plane. The pulmonary artery in this projection, branches into the left pulmonary artery and duct, which connects to the descending aorta. The left atrium lies between the descending and ascending aorta. The flickering foramen ovale flap in the centre of the left atrium in the moving image, often serves to identify the left atrium whatever view of this structure is obtained.

The sections described above display all the connections of the fetal heart which are necessary to identify structural normality. However, many further projections of the heart can be achieved and can be useful in the recognition of normality. Such projections should also be studied and understood in the normal heart as they can prove useful in the elucidation of an abnormality. Figure 1.21b shows a projection of the heart which would not be obtainable postnatally. It is achieved by cutting across the fetal thorax in front of both shoulders (Figure 1.21a). It demonstrates the right atrium and ventricle lying anterior to the ascending aorta, entering the scan plane from the left ventricle behind the plane of section. The pulmonary valve can be seen lying anterior and cranial to the aortic valve. With the ultrasound beam orientated at a slight angle to this plane, the inferior and superior vena cava can be seen entering the right atrium. The right atrial-tricuspid valve connection can also be seen (Figure 1.21c). A further projection of the fetal heart that can be useful is the short axis of left ventricle (Figure 1.22b). This is seen in the long axis of the fetus with the beam in the position seen in Figure 1.22a, i.e. to the left of the sternum and directed towards the left shoulder. The infundibulum of the right ventricle and main pulmonary artery can be seen arching around the left ventricle which is seen as a circle in cross-section. The two ventricles can be seen to 'sit' on the diaphragm.

Figure 1.23 illustrates the orientation of the anterior longitudinal planes with reference to a four-chamber section of the fetal heart. If the heart is approached from the positions 1 to 6 illustrated in Figure 1.5 it can be seen that the beam must be turned through 90°, then moved around the fetal trunk in order to display the sections indicated. This is much easier than it sounds, particularly in the smaller fetus where only a slight tilt of the transducer will produce each plane and when each plane can be imaged in a continuous connecting sequence. In late pregnancy it can be difficult to move round the thorax far enough to produce all the longitudinal planes. It can be seen that the anterior longitudinal sections could be difficult to find if approaching from position 1 in a large fetus, or that the lateral longitudinal sections seen in Figure 1.21a would not be readily found if approaching from position 4. As long as all the cardiac connections are checked it is of no importance which views are used to this purpose.

There are further horizontal views of the fetal thorax which provide information about structural normality of the fetal heart. These must be recognized and understood. Again the important landmark to establish initially is the spine. Once orientated in the four-chamber view, if the transducer is moved cranially the origin of the aorta appears at the crux of the heart. The aorta at its origin is directed towards the right of the thorax going in the opposite direction to the apex. This is seen in Figure 1.24a and the corresponding echocardiogram in Figure 1.24b. Further cranial movement (Figure 1.25a), still maintaining a horizontal section, produces the image seen in Figure 1.25. This is the pulmonary artery connecting through the duct, to the descending aorta. Figure 1.25c is the same view but from a different projection to Figures 1.25a and b. The pulmonary artery, connecting through the duct to the descending aorta just in front of the spine, can be seen. The ascending aorta lies to the right of the main pulmonary artery in each case. Note that the pulmonary valve ring lies almost at right angles to the aortic valve ring (Figure 1.19a).

The pulmonary artery arises from close to the front of the chest, unlike the aorta which arises from the centre of the chest. The pulmonary artery is directed straight back towards the spine, unlike the aorta which sweeps out to the right. Slight angulation and cranial tilt ·from the section seen in Figure 1.25 will produce the image seen in Figure 1.26. The ascending aorta is seen in cross-section, and the main pulmonary artery is seen branching into the right pulmonary artery and the ductus arteriosus. Continuing the horizontal cranial movement allows the arch of the aorta to be seen in the thoracic inlet (Figure 1.27). After the aorta sweeps out to the right it then turns medially to join the descending aorta just to the left of the spine and just above the duct. Angulation between the last two views will allow the duct and arch to be seen in the same projection. Their relative sizes and relationship to each other can be examined (Figures 1.28a,b).

The transducer can be swept up and down these scan planes to recognize each in turn. In the early fetus this will require minimal movement of the transducer and can be accomplished readily. The operator should familiarize himself with each section as it will appear in each possible spinal position. Turning the diagrams and echocardiograms illustrated in Figures 1.23–1.28 through 90, 180 and 270 degrees should help this process. If the spine is always used as an initial reference point when scanning, and the relationship of normal cardiac structures to it is known, the technique of cardiac scanning is soon acquired. Figures 1.29a and 1.29b attempt to illustrate these sections further in diagramatic form. These sections, particularly in the small heart, are much more 'concertina'd' than can be represented diagrammatically.

In whatever section the great arteries are imaged the following points must be noted:

(1) There are two arterial valves, the pulmonary valve anterior and cranial to the aortic valve.
(2) The pulmonary artery is slightly greater than the aorta in size.
(3) The two great arteries are at right angles to each other at their origin.
(4) The aorta arises in the centre of the chest and gives rise to the arch.
(5) The arch gives rise to head and neck vessels.
(6) The pulmonary artery arises from the anterior ventricle and gives rise to the duct.
(7) At least one branch of the pulmonary artery should be seen, the right in horizontal sections, the left in the longitudinal ductal view.

The last projection to be considered in the morphological evaluation of the heart is that of the fetal abdomen. This allows comparison of the relative positions of the abdominal aorta and inferior vena cava. These structures can indicate the atrial situs. Figure 1.30 shows the abdomen in cross-section. Normally the aorta lies on the left of the vertebral body, the inferior vena cava on the right. They are fairly symmetrically positioned. Turning from this position in to the long axis of the fetus the inferior vena cava can be followed to its connection to the right atrium. The aorta can be demonstrated to lie to the left of the inferior vena cava in the long axis plane of the fetus. These relations of the great vessels in the abdomen denote normal atrial situs.

To reiterate in summary, examination of the fetal heart involves systematically checking the connections of the heart – venous-atrial, atrio-ventricular and ventriculo-arterial. The inferior vena cava can be seen in the abdomen and followed to the anterior atrium. Inferior pulmonary veins can be seen to drain to the left atrium in the four-chamber projection. Superior pulmonary veins can be seen in the long axis of the left ventricle. The atrio-ventricular connection is seen in the four-chamber view. The ventriculo-arterial connections can be examined in any of the additional long axis or transverse views described. If all the points are noted in the four-chamber view and points of great artery anatomy are checked, there are few examples of congenital heart disease which would escape detection. The fetal heart can be examined in all the sections described, but not all are necessary for a diagnostic study. There are five longitudinal fetal cuts – two lateral, the tricuspid–pulmonary and venal caval views; and three coronal, the aortic arch, ductal and short axis views of the left ventricle. The coronal views, relative to the whole fetus, are indicated in Figure 1.31. The lateral longitudinal views, with respect to the whole fetus, are indicated in Figure 1.32. There are five horizontal cuts of the fetus illustrated in Figure 1.33 – the abdominal, four-chamber, four-chamber–aortic root, pulmonary artery–duct, and transverse arch. There are three angled slices of the fetal heart which lie between the horizontal and longitudinal – the long axis of left ventricle, the arch–ductal view, and the right pulmonary artery–ductal view (Figure 1.34). Any combination of these views which allows all the connections and points of four-chamber and arterial anatomy to be checked, constitute an adequate fetal echocardiogram.

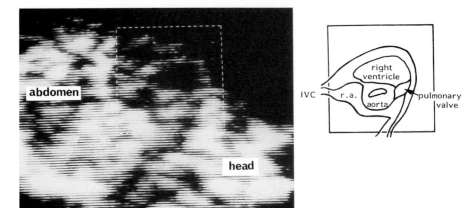

Figure 1.1 Computer assisted sonography allows the tiny fetus of 10 weeks gestation to be seen in surprising detail. The eye sockets of the head can be seen. The arterial connections of the heart can be identified

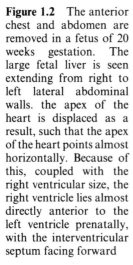

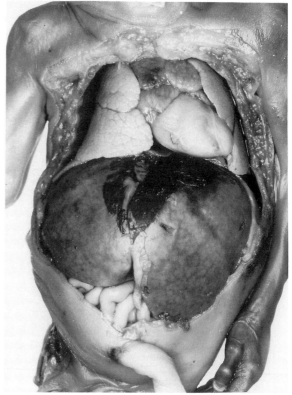

Figure 1.2 The anterior chest and abdomen are removed in a fetus of 20 weeks gestation. The large fetal liver is seen extending from right to left lateral abdominal walls. the apex of the heart is displaced as a result, such that the apex of the heart points almost horizontally. Because of this, coupled with the right ventricular size, the right ventricle lies almost directly anterior to the left ventricle prenatally, with the interventricular septum facing forward

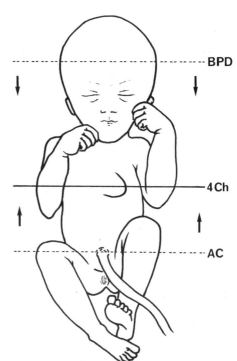

Figure 1.3a The view to achieve   the   abdominal   circumference   is   seen   drawn
straight across the abdomen.
The   view   to   achieve   the
biparietal diameter is straight
across the largest dimension of
the head. Moving between these
sections the four-chamber view
of the heart will be seen cutting
horizontally across the thorax
just above the diaphragm

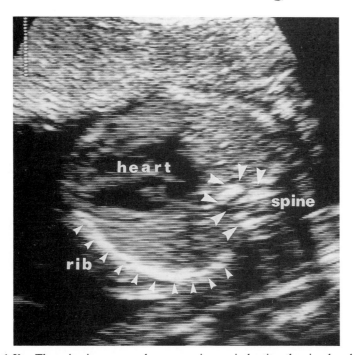

Figure 1.3b   The spine is seen as a bony prominence indenting the circular shape of
the thorax. If one rib is seen complete, as here, then the operator can be sure of the
correct horizontal plane. The heart can be seen in the anterior thorax

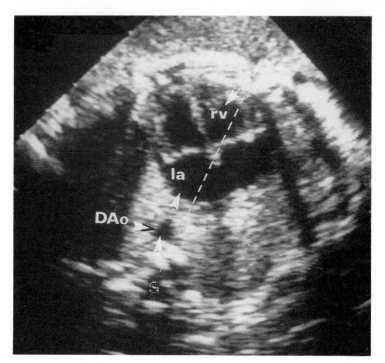

Figure 1.4 However the transverse section of the fetal thorax lies relative to the transducer, the method of orientation is always the same. The spine is first located. The anterior chest wall or sternum lies opposite the spine. The right ventricle lies beneath the sternum. Returning to the spine, the descending aorta is seen as a circular structure slightly to the left of the spine. The left atrium lies immediately anterior to the descending aorta

Figure 1.5 The cross-section of the fetal thorax is represented diagramatically. The fetus may lie with its spine in any orientation around a 360° circle to the transducer but basically there are six principal positions. The four-chamber view will appear different when the beam is parallel to the ventricular septum, as in positions 1 and 3, than when the beam is perpendicular to the septum as in positions 2 and 4. Position 5 will have an appearance between those seen in positions 3 and 4. Approaching the fetus with the spine in position 6, the fetal heart may be completely shadowed by the spine. The operator must then move around the fetal thorax, or maternal abdomen, to approach from positions 1 or 2

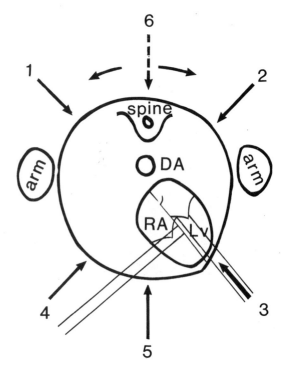

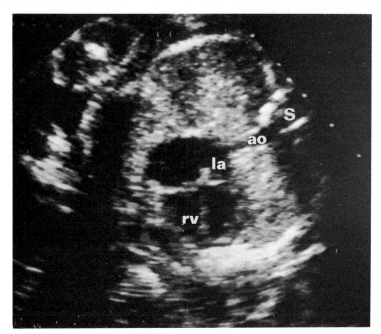

Figure 1.6 The fetal heart is approached from the right back (position 1). The ultrasound beam is almost parallel to the septum. The crux of the heart is seen clearly. the commonly observed 'fading' of the ventricular septum just below the atrioventricular valves is seen

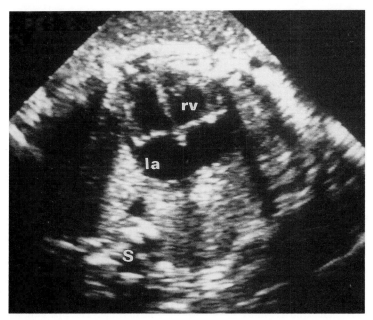

Figure 1.7 The four-chamber view is here approached almost directly from the apex or left anterior chest with the beam parallel to the septum (position 3). The image is identical to Figure 1.6 except inverted antero-superiorly. Because the heart is closer to the transducer in position 3 than in position 1 the image is more clear

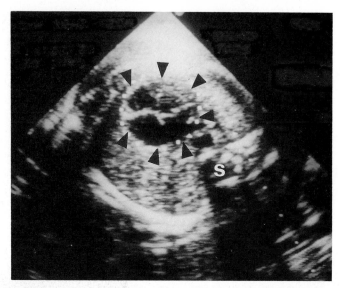

Figure 1.8   Examination of the crux of the heart shows the differential insertion of the septal cusps of the atrioventricular valves. The tricuspid insertion is slightly more apical than the mitral insertion. The heart occupies approximately one third of the fetal thorax (arrows)

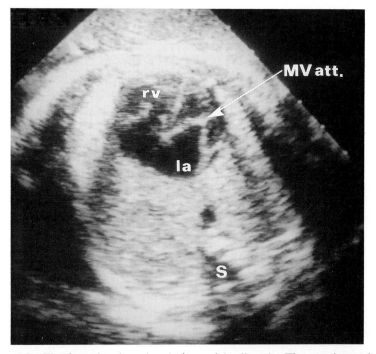

Figure 1.9   The four-chamber view is imaged in diastole. The opening atrioventricular valves can be seen. The normal chordal attachment of each valve can often be seen. The mitral valve is attached to the posterior left ventricular wall only, whereas the tricuspid valve is attached to the septum and posterior wall

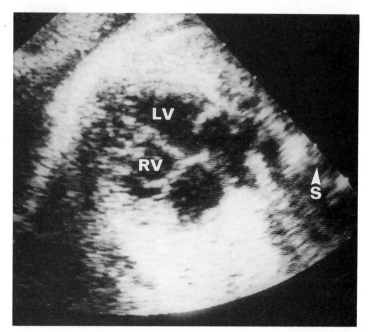

Figure 1.10 The fetal heart is approached from the left back (position 2). The beam is almost perpendicular to the ventricular septum. The left ventricle is closest to the transducer. Wall and septal thicknesses are clearly defined. The septum in this view can be seen to be intact to the crux of the heart

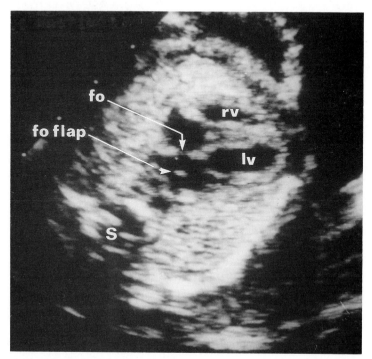

Figure 1.11 The heart is imaged from the anterior right chest wall (position 4). The right ventricle is closer to the transducer. The margins of the foramen ovale can be defined and the flap valve can be seen lying within the cavity of the left atrium. This view can be seen to be the same as Figure 1.10 but antero-superiorly inverted

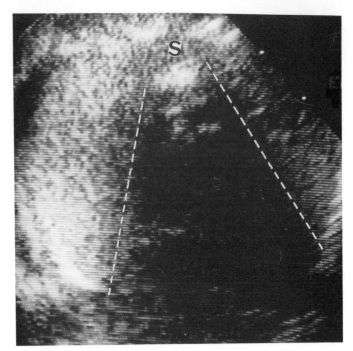

Figure 1.12 The spine lies directly below the transducer, producing a wedge-shaped shadow completely obscuring the heart

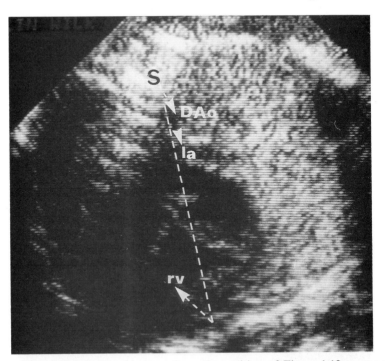

Figure 1.13 Moving the transducer from the position of Figure 1.12 to one side produces an image from position 1. Although the spine still shadows part of the heart, by using the method of orientation from the spine described above, structures can be identified. Two atria and the crux of the heart can be examined. To examine the ventricles the spinal shadow would need to be swung to the other side by moving the transducer to position 2

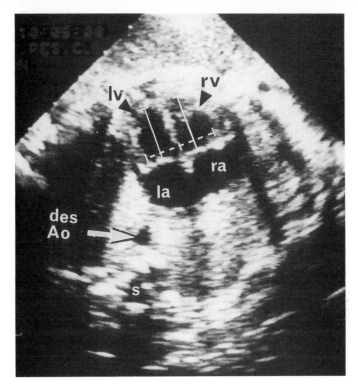

Figure 1.14 In the four-chamber view two atria of approximately equal size are seen. The lengths and widths of the two ventricles just below the atrioventricular valves are similar

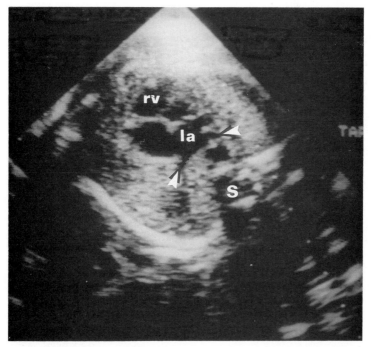

Figure 1.15 The heart is imaged in the four-chamber view. The inferior pulmonary veins can be seen entering the left atrium. They are outlined passing into lung substance by the fluid-filled lung tissue

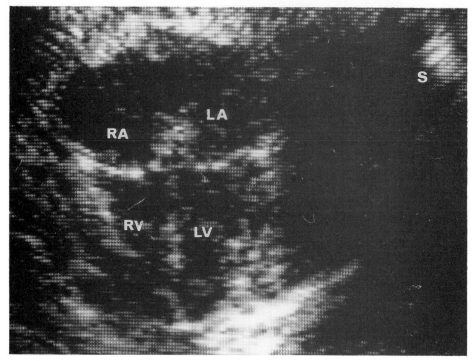

Figure 1.16a The heart is seen in the four-chamber projection. Shadowing from a rib lies between the spine and the heart

Figure 1.16b Moving cranially from the position in Figure 1.16a allows the aortic root arising from the left ventricle to be imaged in the centre of the heart

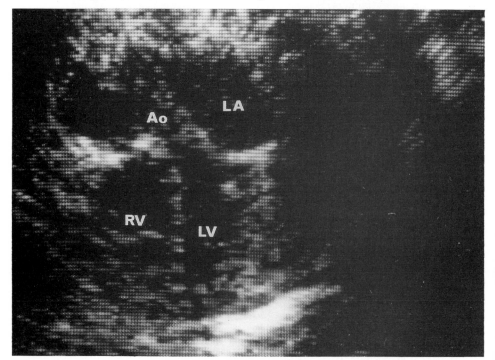

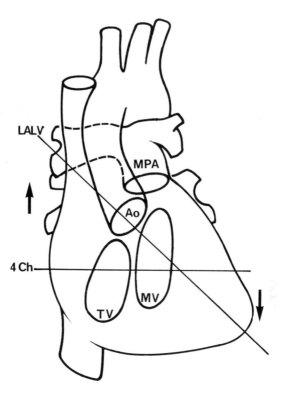

Figure 1.17a The ultrasound beam is angled from the transverse four-chamber plane to visualize the left ventricle in long axis. The beam passes through the mitral valve, the aortic valve and a superior pulmonary vein

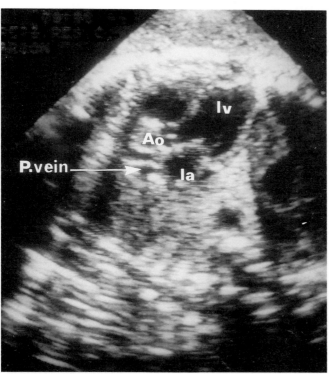

Figure 1.17b The fetal heart is imaged in the long axis of the left ventricle. The left heart connections can be seen in this view from pulmonary veins to left atrium, via the mitral valve to left ventricle, to the aorta. Aortic-mitral and aortic-septal continuity can be noted

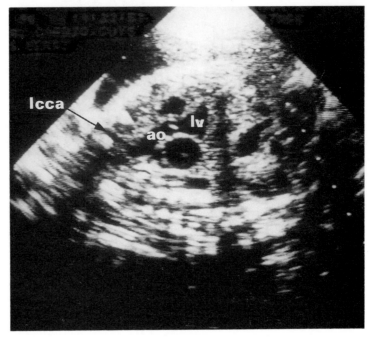

Figure 1.18 The ascending aorta is followed from the left ventricle to the beginning of the arch from which the first head vessel can be seen to arise

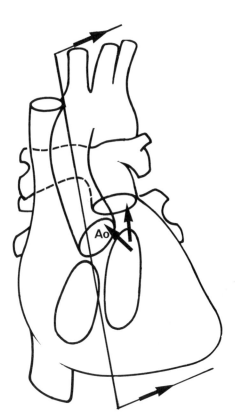

Figure 1.19a The ultrasound beam is angled into the heart from the centre of the anterior chest towards the left back. The beam is longitudinal to the fetus almost parallel to the spine. Note that the pulmonary valve ring lies almost at right angles to the aortic valve ring within the heart (arrows)

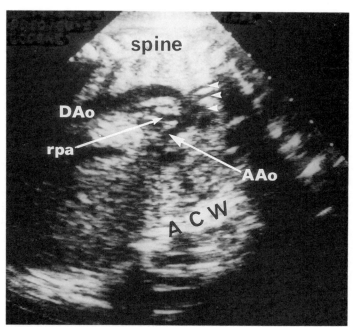

Figure 1.19b The arch of the aorta is seen, with head and neck vessels arising from it. The arch forms a tight hook with the ascending aorta tucking into the centre of the chest. The right pulmonary artery lies within the hook. The descending aorta lies almost parallel and anterior to the spine.

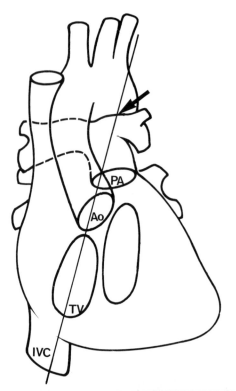

Figure 1.20a The transducer beam transects the inferior vena cava, tricuspid valve, aorta, and pulmonary artery. The duct lies at the point of junction between the main pulmonary artery and the underside of the arch (arrow)

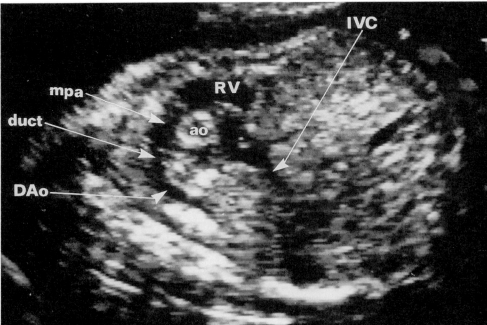

Figure 1.20b The fetus is cut in a longitudinal plane. The inferior vena cava, tricuspid valve, pulmonary valve and duct are all seen. The aorta is seen in cross-section in the centre of the scan plane. The duct connects to the descending aorta posteriorly

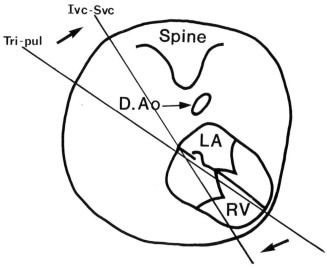

Figure 1.21a The ultrasound beam cuts the fetus in a longitudinal plane. The orientation of the tricuspid pulmonary and IVC–SVC planes to the four-chamber view are seen here

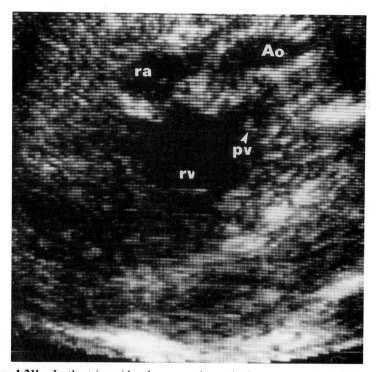

Figure 1.21b In the tricuspid pulmonary plane, the beam cuts across the anterior thorax between the shoulders, just in front of the right side of the ventricular septum. The tricuspid valve is transected, as is the aorta sweeping out of the left ventricle anteriorly into the plane of section

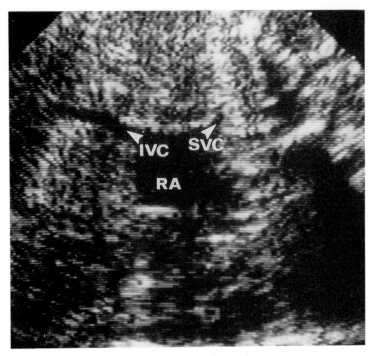

Figure 1.21c   Posterior angulation from the section in Figure 1.21b will show an image where the superior and inferior vena cava are entering the right atrium opposite or directly infero-superior to each other

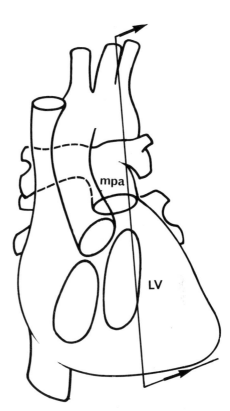

Figure 1.22a The beam is directed from the left side of the sternum towards the left shoulder, almost parallel to the coronal plane of the fetus. The beam cuts the left ventricle in short axis. The infundibulum of the right ventricle and pulmonary valve lie anterior to the left ventricle

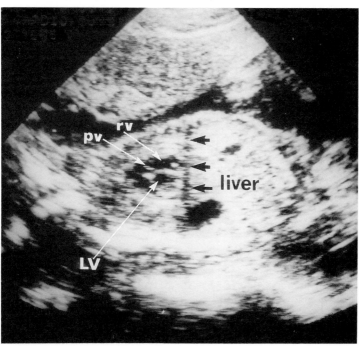

Figure 1.22b The two ventricles are seen 'sitting' on the diaphragm (arrows). The left ventricle is a circular posterior structure. The right ventricle, pulmonary outflow tract and pulmonary valve are anterior to the left ventricle

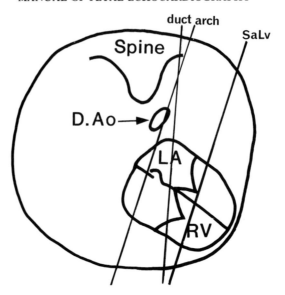

Figure 1.23   The three anterior longitudinal scan planes are illustrated with reference to a four-chamber view. The arch view is achieved with oblique angulation across the chest, the ductal view more or less with direct antero-posterior angulation. The short axis of left ventricle is again an angled plane across the left side of the thorax

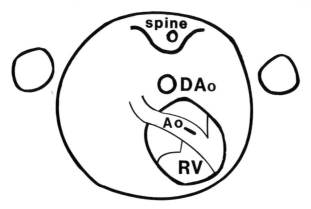

Figure 1.24a   The transducer is moved cranially but horizontally from the four-chamber view to image the origin of the aorta from the left ventricle

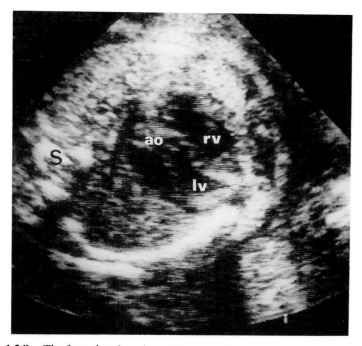

Figure 1.24b   The four-chamber view with the origin of the aorta at the crux of the heart is seen. Note that the echocardiogram needs to be turned through 90° and laterally inverted to match the drawing. The operator must learn to interpret the images whatever the relative fetal and spinal positions

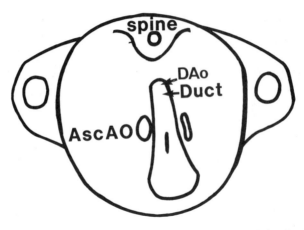

Figure 1.25a A horizontal section of the thorax at the level of the shoulders allows the ductus arteriosus to be seen connecting the main pulmonary artery to the descending aorta

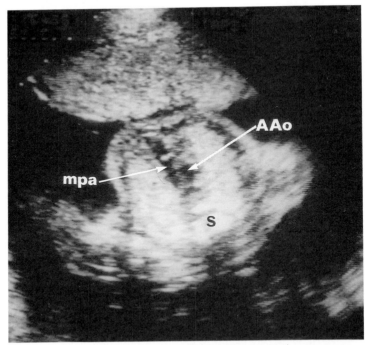

Figure 1.25b With the spine in the opposite position from the above diagram but in the same section the same features can be noted. The pulmonary artery arises from the front of the chest and is directed posteriorly towards the spine. The ascending aorta lies to the right of the main pulmonary artery

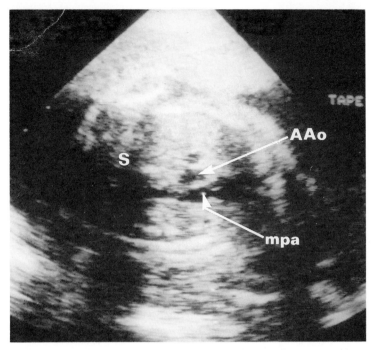

Figure 1.25c   This is again the same section as the previous two figures but from a different projection. The pulmonary outflow tract passes from the right to the left of the picture. The spinal shadow obscures the ductal-descending aorta junction

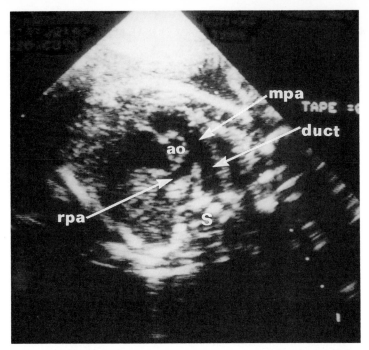

Figure 1.26 The transducer is tilted from the sections seen Figures 1.25b and 1.25c to visualize the branching of the main pulmonary artery into right pulmonary artery and ductus arteriosus. The duct joins the descending aorta just anterior to the spine

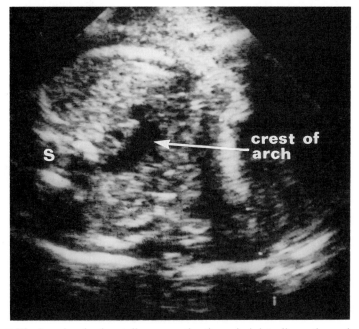

Figure 1.27 Imaging horizontally across the thoracic inlet allows the arch of the aorta to be seen. The ductus will lie just below this section and the transducer can be swept between the two views, to compare the size of the vessels and their relative orientation. The pulmonary artery-ductus lies to the left of the aortic arch in the fetal chest

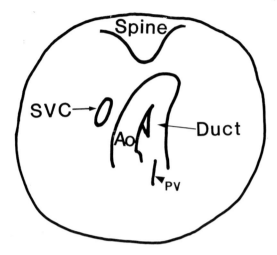

Figure 1.28a   An angled view across the thoracic inlet allows the arch and duct to be seen in the same section. Their relative sizes and relationship can be noted. The superior vena cava will lie to the right of the transverse arch in the fetal thorax

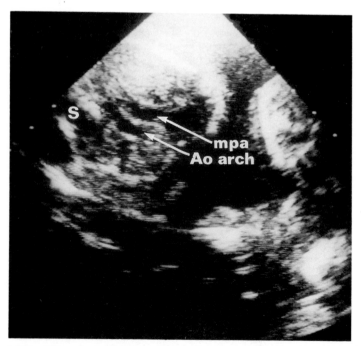

Figure 1.28b   The echocardiogram shows the crest of the aortic arch and main pulmonary artery ductal connection where they both communicate with the descending aorta

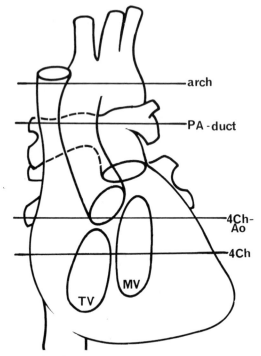

Figure 1.29a The heart is viewed from the front with the four horizontal planes indicated. The first or lowest section shows the four-chamber view, the next the four-chamber–aortic root view. Moving further cranially the pulmonary artery-ductal connection is seen, just below the crest of the aortic arch

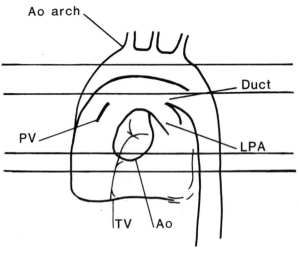

Figure 1.29b The heart is viewed from the side with the same four horizontal planes drawn

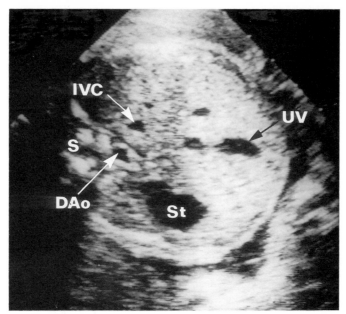

Figure 1.30   The abdomen is sectioned transversely at the level of the umbilical vein. The stomach lies in the left of the abdomen. The aorta is seen, pulsating in the moving image, anterior and to the left of the spine. The inferior vena cava lies slightly anterior to the aorta on the right side of the abdomen

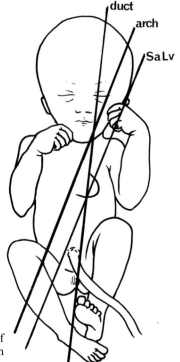

Figure 1.31   The longitudinal anterior sections of
the fetus are displayed, to image the duct, the arch
and the left ventricle in short axis

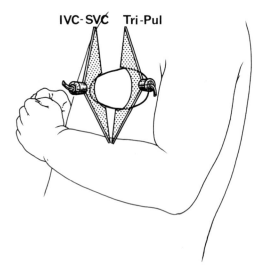

Figure 1.32   The fetus is imaged from the side. The planes of transducer orientation
necessary to image the two lateral longitudinal planes, the tricuspid pulmonary and
the inferior–superior vena caval planes, are indicated

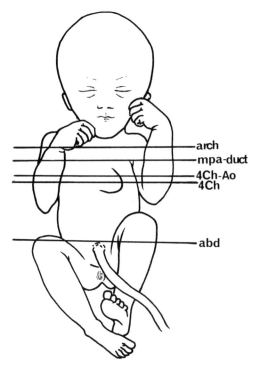

Figure 1.33 The horizontal cuts of the fetus to view the abdomen, the four chambers, the four-chamber–aortic root, the main pulmonary artery-ductal connection and the aortic arch are indicated

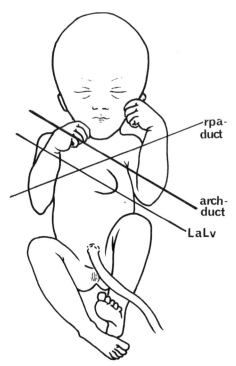

Figure 1.34 The angled views are indicated. These image the left ventricle in long axis, the arch-duct in the same section, and the right pulmonary artery-ductal view

CHAPTER 2

Normal fetal cardiac anatomy – the M-mode echocardiogram

M-mode echocardiography has an important role in the evaluation of fetal cardiac abnormality and fetal arrhythmias. Experience of the technique of M-mode should be gained first of all, however, in the normal fetal heart. Our initial measurements of intracardiac structures were all acquired using M-mode tracings. This was firstly because M-mode can define intracardiac surfaces more precisely than a frozen cross-sectional image. Also, measurements could be timed more accurately within the cardiac cycle. Measurement data could be directly compared with postnatal data which was all based on M-mode echocardiography.

The heart must first be evaluated by cross-sectional examination to locate the structures to be studied. Two projections of the heart are necessary for measurement data – the short axis of left ventricle and the ductal view in the coronal plane of the fetus. For the first (Figure 2.1), the M line is positioned through the right and left ventricles at right angles to the ventricular septum. This projection is chosen for several reasons. First, it is similar to the position in which M-mode is performed postnatally and measurements can be made in the same place in the ventricles. Second, the beam must be perpendicular to the septum if errors in measuring the ventricular cavities are to be avoided. Third, this view of the fetal heart is nearly always readily obtainable whatever the fetal lie. The tracing achieved in this position is seen in Figure 2.2. From this tracing septal and posterior left ventricular wall thickness, and right and left ventricular internal dimensions in systole and diastole can be measured. The normal ranges for these measurements throughout gestation are seen in Figures 2.3–2.6. An important point to note is that the ventricular septum moves in the same way as postnatally i.e. septum moves towards the posterior left ventricular wall in systole. This is more clearly seen in Figure 2.7. Paradoxical septal motion does not occur in the fetus if recordings are made in the correct position. This contradicts an early suggestion that this was a common finding in the fetus[22].

The second section for obtaining fetal cardiac measurements (Figure 2.8) is the ductal view of the heart in the coronal section of the fetus. The M line is positioned through the aorta in short axis at its origin and the left atrium. The tracing achieved in this position is seen in Figure 2.9. The growth of these structures throughout pregnancy is seen in Figures 2.10 and 2.11.

It is important to interpret these measurements in context both with each other and within the setting of the individual fetus. Our cardiac measurements were acquired in fetuses dated by early biparietal diameter measurements. In a growth-retarded fetus all the cardiac measurements will be relatively low for the gestational age. Conversely, one cardiac measurement out of step with the others and the state of fetal growth may indicate a structural cardiac abnormality.

Examination of the motion of each cardiac valve can also be recorded, but this has little practical usefulness. Doppler analysis is a more accurate and informative method of valvular evaluation and has largely superseded qualitative and quantitative M-mode echocardiography.

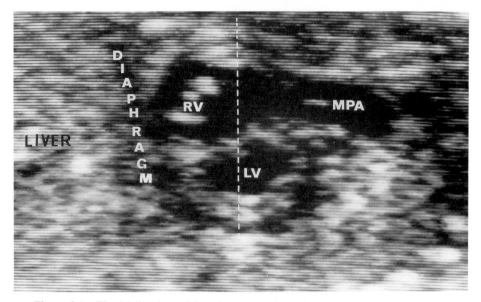

Figure 2.1 The M-line is positioned through the left ventricle when imaged in a short axis projection. The left ventricle can be seen contracting concentrically in the moving image. The right ventricle is seen as a tube arteriorly with the pulmonary valve at the cranial end. Trabeculation can be seen in the apex of the right ventricle. The two ventricles lie on the diaphragm with the liver to the left of the picture. The M-line is perpendicular to the intraventricular septum

M–MODE THROUGH BOTH VENTRICLES

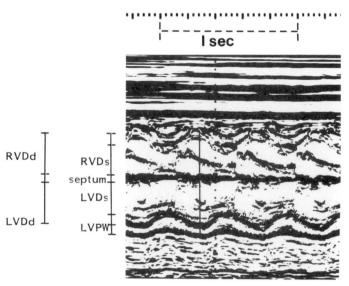

Figure 2.2 With the M-line positioned as in Figure 2.1 this recording is achieved. Measurements of right and left ventricular cavities in systole and diastole, septal and posterior left ventricular wall thickness can be made

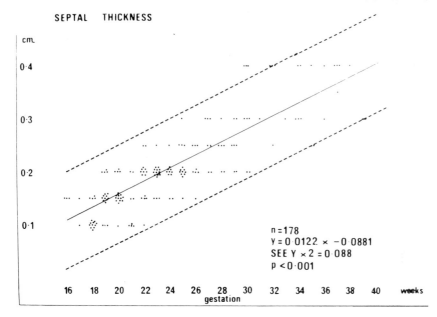

Figure 2.3   The increasing thickness of the septal wall is plotted against gestational age

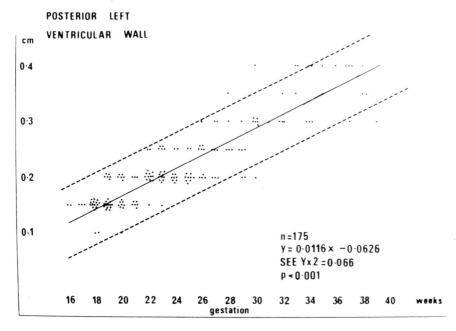

Figure 2.4   The posterior left ventricular wall thickness in diastole is plotted against gestational age. It can be seen to be similar in thickness to the ventricular septum

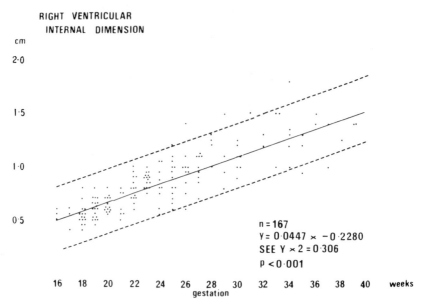

Figure 2.5   The right ventricular cavity increases steadily throughout pregnancy. In this projection it has a similar size to the left ventricle

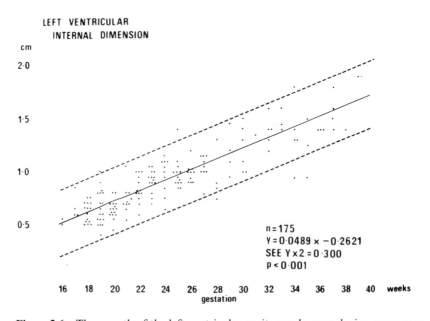

Figure 2.6   The growth of the left ventricular cavity can be seen during pregnancy

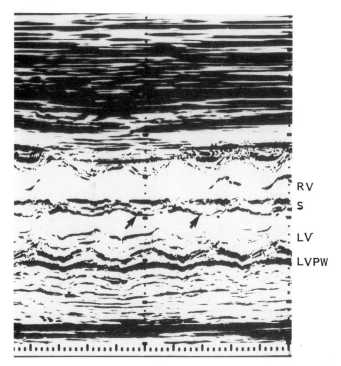

Figure 2.7 The septum in the normal fetus moves towards the left ventricle (arrows) when the mitral valve closes. This is the same as in postnatal life. The recording should be made just below the mitral valve leaflets. This recording was made at 24 weeks gestation

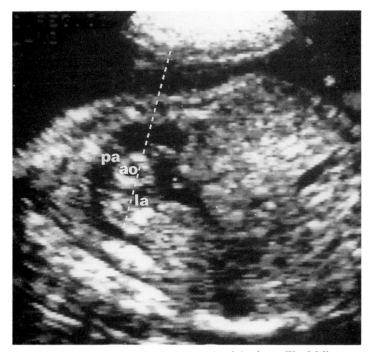

Figure 2.8 The ductus is imaged in the long axis of the fetus. The M-line crosses the right ventricle, the aorta and left atrium

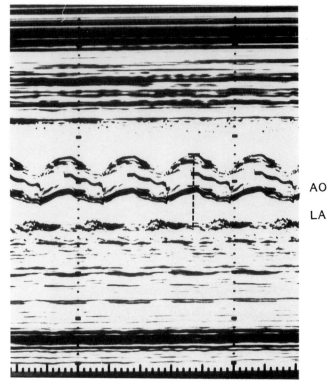

AO

LA

Figure 2.9   The tracing achieved with the M-line positioned as in Figure 2.8 is seen. The left atrial and aortic root measurements are made, from leading edge to leading edge, in diastole

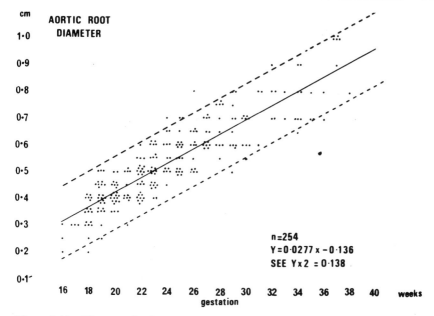

Figure 2.10   The growth of the aortic root throughout pregnancy is seen

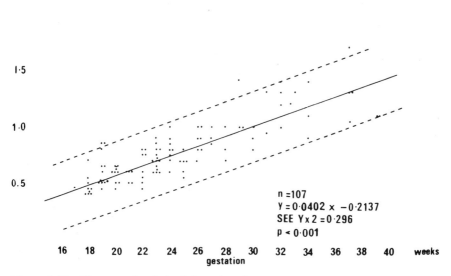

Figure 2.11   The growth of the left atrium is seen throughout pregnancy. It is consistently larger in size than the aortic root

CHAPTER 3

Normal fetal cardiac anatomy – Doppler echocardiography

Doppler is an extremely useful addition to the cross-sectional echocardiographic study. Each cardiac valve can be interrogated and normal characteristics of blood flow velocity observed. The smallest sample volume possible for the machine used is placed in the cavity of each ventricle imaged in the four-chamber view. This will display the velocity of blood flow through the tricuspid or mitral valves. The direction of blood flow should be less than 20° from the angle of the Doppler beam. The four-chamber view as imaged from positions 1 and 3 in Figure 1.5 are suitable. If the fetus is lying such that the four-chamber view is only seen from positions 2 or 4 the angle of Doppler insonation will be unsuitable. The operator must wait for the fetus to move, or try to move as far round the thorax as possible to achieve a better angle, or abandon interrogation of the atrioventricular valves. Only in rare circumstances will the information required from atrioventricular valve interrogation not be obtainable from arterial valve examination. Usually the most important flow calculation to make is relative R/L estimate of flow and this can be measured at either the atrioventricular or the arterial valves. The correct orientation and a representative tracing of tricuspid valve are seen in Figures 3.1a and b. The corresponding image and tracing for the mitral valve is seen in Figures 3.2a and b. It can be seen that on the mitral tracing there is commonly a small systolic jet in the opposite direction from the mitral jet. This is because the sample volume, which is relatively large at 2 mm compared to the cavity of the fetal left ventricle, overlaps the outflow tract. This can be minimized by placing the sample volume as close to the ventricular wall as possible, but as it is not included in calculations of blood flow it is of little importance.

It should be noted that the atrioventricular valves have a characteristic double peak of blood flow. The passive filling phase is less than the active atrial phase which forms the second peak. The passive filling phase increases with fetal breathing. An example of a tracing recorded during breathing is seen in Figure 3.3. The passive filling phase also increases with gestation so that by the end of pregnancy the atrioventricular valve blood flow velocity tracing has the appearance seen in Figure 3.4. The maximum velocity of tricuspid valve flow does not change with gestation and is a mean of $51.95 \pm 19.4 \, \text{cm s}^{-1}$ (2 SD). The maximum velocity of mitral blood flow does not change with gestation and is $48.49 \pm 20.8 \, \text{cm s}^{-1}$ (2 SD). Mean temporal velocity of each valve is obtained by planimetering the area underneath the spectral velocity display throughout the cardiac cycle and dividing by the time over which the flow was traced. Velocities are traced along the zero line during systole. An average of three beats are used. Tracings showing the variation in pattern associated with fetal breathing are not used for mean velocity calculations. Mean velocity of tricuspid valve flow is $13.5 \pm 6 \, \text{cm s}^{-1}$ (2 SD); mean velocity of mitral valve flow is $12.5 \pm 5.2 \, \text{cm s}^{-1}$ (2 SD).

Transvalvular flow can be calculated from the formula[23,24].

$$\text{flow} = (\text{angle corrected mean velocity}) \times \text{area.}$$

The Hewlett Packard automatically corrects for angle. With some equipment this needs to be calculated and included in the equation. The area of the valve orifice is calculated by multiplying the radius^2 by π. This assumes a circular orifice for both atrioventricular valves which may be inaccurate. Also the measurement of the fibrous ring of the valves in diastole can be difficult to make accurately. This can introduce a substantial error into absolute flow measurements. However, with these reservations flow measurements are probably fairly close to real values. Tricuspid orifice size is consistently slightly greater than mitral; mean tricuspid velocity similar to or slightly greater than mitral. Growth charts for diameter measurements throughout pregnancy are seen for the tricuspid and mitral valves in Figures 3.5a and 3.6a, with the methods of measurement illustrated in Figures 3.5b and 3.6b respectively. Tricuspid flow is consistently higher than mitral flow. It should be appreciated that diurnal and individual variations of normal blood flow are quite wide. Absolute blood flow through the tricuspid valve rises throughout pregnancy from about $50 \, \text{ml min}^{-1}$ at 17/52 gestation to approximately $800 \, \text{ml min}^{-1}$ at term. Flow through the mitral valve rises from about $30 \, \text{ml min}^{-1}$ at 17/52 to about $600 \, \text{ml min}^{-1}$ at term. Figures 3.7 and

3.8 show the blood flow through the tricuspid valve and mitral valves plotted against gestational age. The ratio of TV/MV flow throughout pregnancy ranges from 0.8 to 1.8 in the normal heart.

It is important when atrioventricular valve regurgitation is suspected to position the sample volume in each atrium close to the valve. Normally there should only be forward flow through the valve in diastole with no back flow during systole. Atrioventricular valve regurgitation should be suspected if there are differential atrial sizes.

Evaluation of the arterial blood flow velocity can be made in a similar fashion to atrioventricular valve interrogation. It is usually easy to place the sample volume in the pulmonary artery in the correct orientation and this is illustrated in Figure 3.9a with the resultant trace in Figure 3.9b. It can be difficult to achieve a good angle on the aorta but it is possible with practice. A suitable position is shown in Figure 3.10a with the resultant tracing in Figure 3.10b. In the arterial tracing of flow velocity there is one peak with a sharp rise to peak as illustrated. This acceleration time is similar for both arterial valves, suggesting equal or similar pressures on both sides of the fetal heart. The mean velocity is obtained in the same way as for the atrioventricular valves by planimetering under the spectral display and recording zero flow in diastole. The mean velocity in the pulmonary valve is $17.2 \pm 8.0 \, \text{cm s}^{-1}$ (2 SD), and in the aortic valve $18.0 \pm 8.6 \, \text{cm s}^{-1}$ (2 SD).

Measurement of the arterial valve orifices is easier and more accurate than that of the atrioventricular valves. The walls of the great artery can be imaged more clearly such that the internal diameter can be precisely resolved. The measurement is made in diastole at the site of the closed arterial valve. The method of measurement of each valve is seen in Figures 3.11a and 3.12a. The diameter of the pulmonary artery and aorta is plotted against gestation in Figures 3.11b and 3.12b. The pulmonary artery is consistently larger than the aorta, although the mean velocity of flow through the aorta may be slightly greater than through the pulmonary artery. The calculated blood flow is from about $20 \, \text{mL min}^{-1}$ at 17/52 through both the pulmonary artery and the aorta, rising to approximately $700 \, \text{mL min}^{-1}$ through the pulmonary artery at term, and $500 \, \text{mL min}^{-1}$ through the aorta. The pulmonary blood flow is usually 60% of the combined cardiac output but a range of 50–70% is normal. The values for blood flow through the aorta and pulmonary artery are plotted against gestational age in Figures 3.13 and 3.14. Although blood flow through the aorta and mitral valve should be the same for any given patient at each gestational age it can be seen that blood flow is slightly greater if the atrioventricular valve is used to estimate flow. The case is similar with pulmonary and tricuspid valve flow estimates. This is perhaps because the atrioventricular valve measurements are difficult to make accurate and reproducible. For this reason we prefer to quantitate aortic and pulmonary blood flow and feel that these values are more precise. Examination of the graphs (Figures 3.13 and 3.14) shows that at 26 weeks gestation the combined cardiac output is approximately $450\,\mathrm{mL\,min^{-1}}$. The average fetal weight is 1 kg at this gestation. Thus, the combined output is $450\,\mathrm{mL\,min^{-1}\,kg^{-1}}$ at this gestation: 250 mL through the right heart, and 200 mL through the left heart.

In summary, a lot of useful normal information can be derived from the Doppler study. Forward flow, normal pattern, velocity and volume through each cardiac valve can be identified and recorded.

Another method of Doppler evaluation that has proved helpful is the A/B ratio of the waveform in the umbilical artery. Figure 3.15 illustrates the method, and Figure 3.16 a normal trace at 24 weeks gestation. The normal range for systolic to diastolic ratio has been established throughout pregnancy[25,26]. An abnormal recording will indicate a poor prognosis (Figure 3.17). In particular, absence of diastolic flow in our experience has always been followed by intrauterine death within the ensuing 1–2 weeks in pregnancies which continue. In appropriate circumstances with adequate maturity this sign is an indication for delivery.

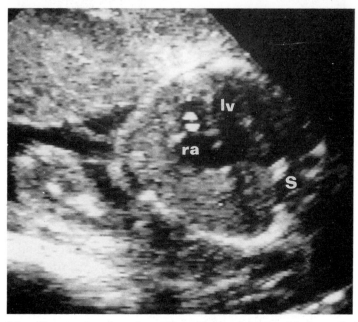

Figure 3.1a The sample volume is positioned in the right ventricle just apical to the tricuspid leaflets

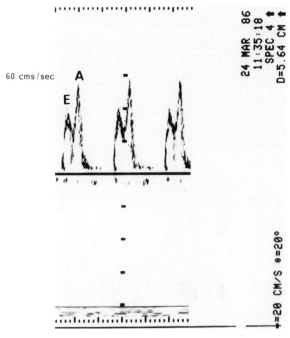

Figure 3.1b The tracing achieved with the sample volume positioned as in Figure 3.1a. The passive filling phase (E) is less than the active filling phase (A). The maximum velocity in this case is around 60 cm s^{-1}

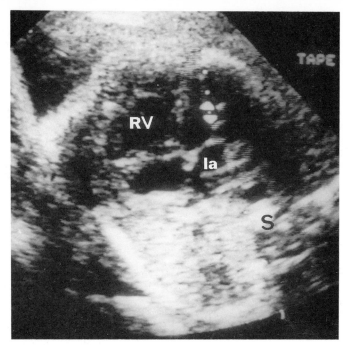

Figure 3.2a The sample volume is positioned in the left ventricle. The direction of blood flow is almost directly towards the transducer

VELOCITY OF BLOOD FLOW
THROUGH MITRAL VALVE −22/52

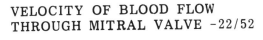

40cm / sec

flow
thro'
MV

flow
in
LVOT

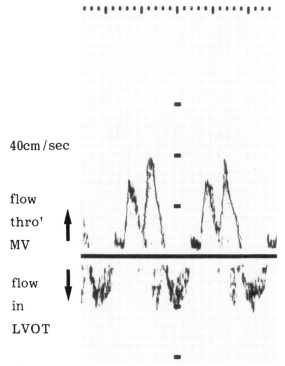

Figure 3.2b The tracing achieved when the sample volume is positioned as in Figure 3.2a. Maximum velocity in this patient is about $40\,\mathrm{cm\,s^{-1}}$. There is some flow in the left ventricular outflow tract recorded in this tracing

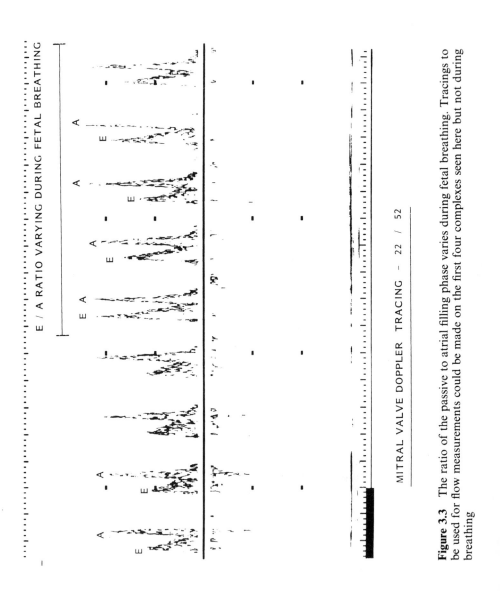

Figure 3.3 The ratio of the passive to atrial filling phase varies during fetal breathing. Tracings to be used for flow measurements could be made on the first four complexes seen here but not during breathing

VELOCITY OF BLOOD FLOW THROUGH

TRICUSPID VALVE – 40 weeks

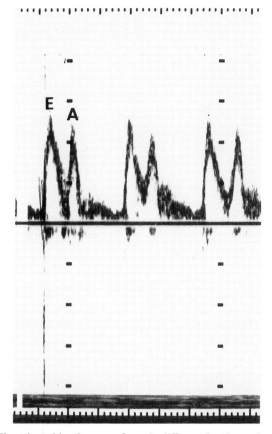

Figure 3.4   The tricuspid valve waveform is different by the end of the pregnancy. The E wave is equal to or greater than the A wave. After birth the E wave is always much greater than the A wave

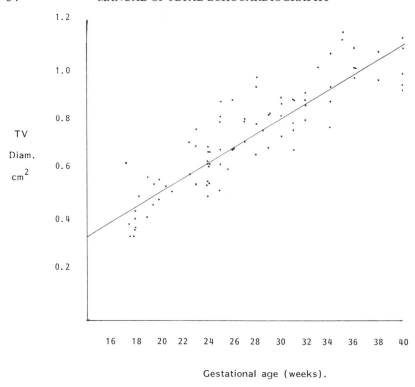

TV

Diam.

cm^2

Gestational age (weeks).

Figure 3.5a The diameter of the tricuspid valve is measured as seen below. The growth is plotted against gestation. There is a fairly wide scatter of results reflecting the difficulty of accurate measurement

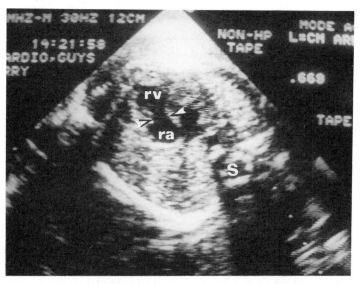

Figure 3.5b The heart is imaged in the four-chamber view. The fibrous ring of the tricuspid valve can be measured as indicated in diastole

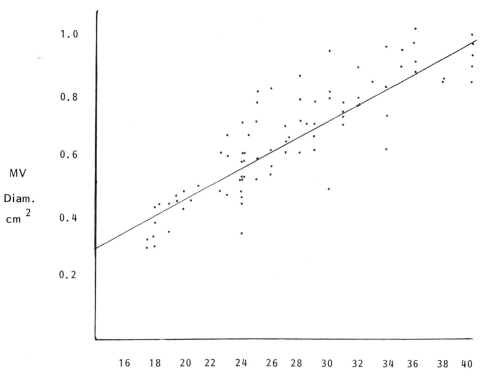

Figure 3.6a   The measurement of the mitral valve orifice is plotted against gestational age. Again there is a wide scatter of normal values

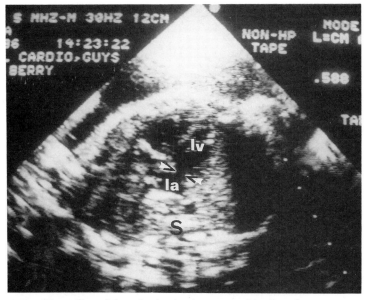

Figure 3.6b   The orifice of the mitral valve is measured in diastole

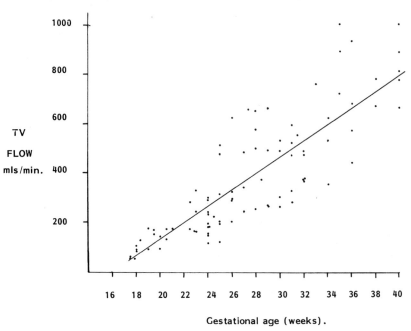

Figure 3.7 The tricuspid valve flow is plotted against gestational age. There is a fairly wide scatter of results particularly in the last 12 weeks of pregnancy

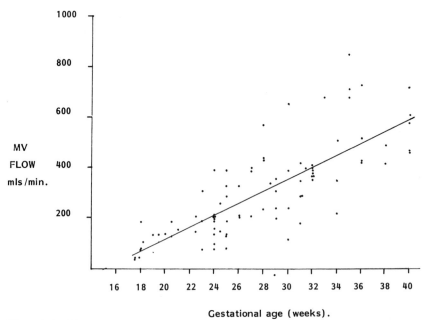

Figure 3.8 The mitral valve flow is plotted against gestational age from 17 weeks to term

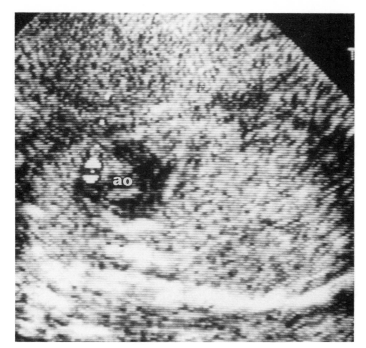

Figure 3.9a The pulmonary artery is imaged in the long axis of the fetus in the ductal plane. The sample volume can be positioned just beyond the pulmonary valve. The direction of flow is almost directly in line with the sample volume

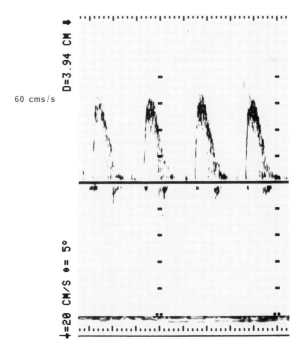

Figure 3.9b The waveform of pulmonary artery flow is seen (here at 24 weeks gestation). There is a fast rise to peak velocity. Maximum velocity here is just over $60\,\mathrm{cm/s^{-1}}$

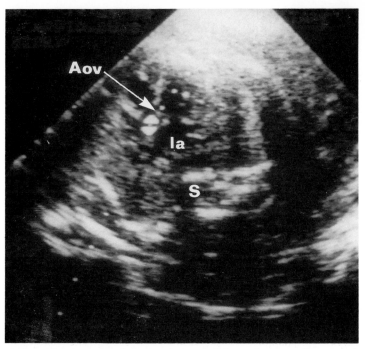

Figure 3.10a The four-chamber view is imaged from the apex. The transducer is then angled cranially to visualize the origin of the aorta. The sample volume is then positioned just beyond the aortic valve. The direction of flow is almost in line with the sample volume

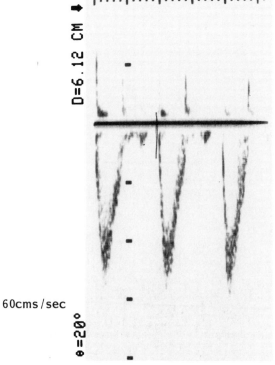

Figure 3.10b The velocity of blood flow through the aorta (here at 22 weeks gestation) is seen to be approximately $50\,\mathrm{cm\,s^{-1}}$ at the maximum point

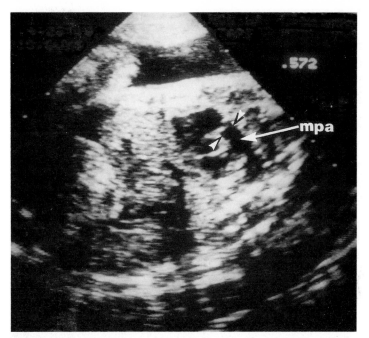

Figure 3.11a The pulmonary artery is imaged here in the ductal plane. The measurement of the internal diameter of the pulmonary artery is made at the upper end of the pulmonary valve in diastole

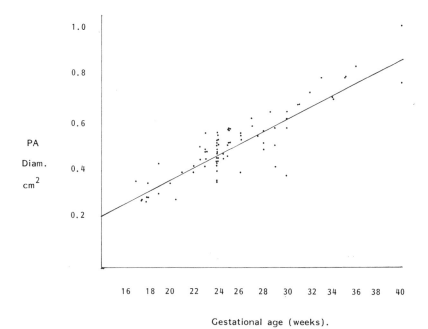

Figure 3.11b The diameter of the pulmonary valve is plotted against gestational age. The ease of making this measurement precisely is reflected in the narrow scatter of results

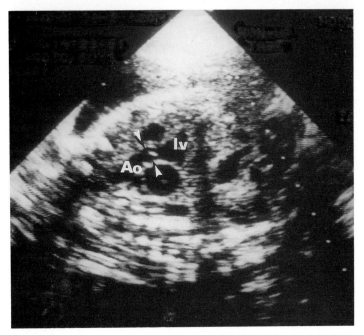

Figure 3.12a   The aorta is imaged in the long axis of the left ventricle. The calipers are positioned to measure the ascending aorta in diastole

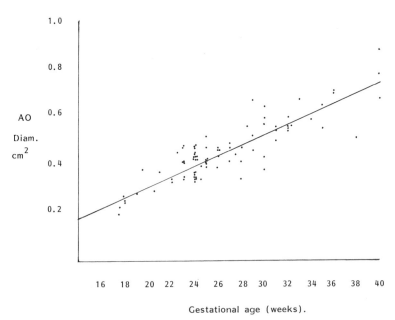

Figure 3.12b   The diameter of the aorta is plotted against the gestational age. Again, measurements are fairly closely grouped around the mean

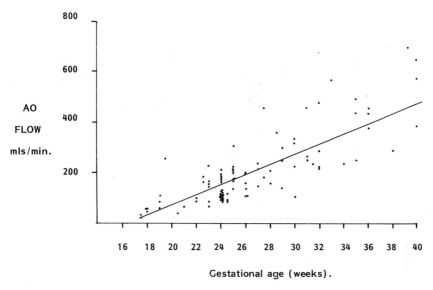

Figure 3.13   The blood flow estimated in the aorta is plotted against gestational age. It can be seen that pulmonary blood flow is consistently slightly greater than aortic

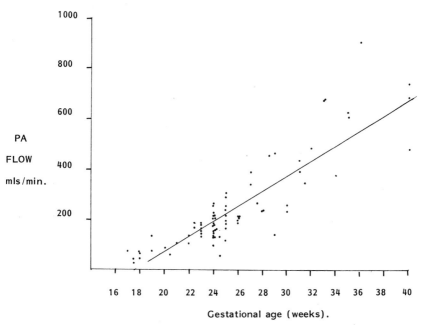

Figure 3.14   The calculated pulmonary artery blood flow is plotted against gestational age

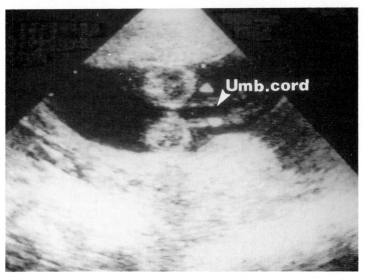

Figure 3.15 The umbilical cord is visualized floating in the amniotic fluid. The sample volume size is increased to cover the whole of the cord

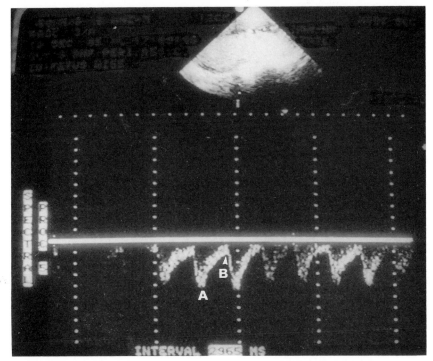

Figure 3.16 A normal tracing of the umbilical waveform is seen at 24 weeks gestation. The A/B ratio is approximately 3:1 which is within normal limits

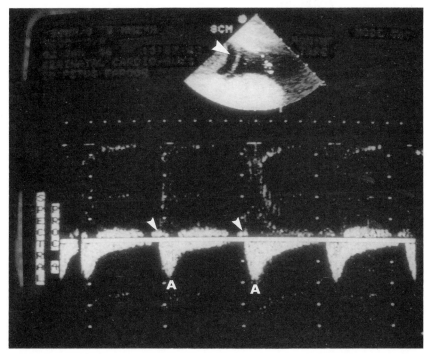

Figure 3.17 The Doppler sample volume is positioned in the umbilical cord. There is fetal ascites (large arrow). There is a bradycardia of less than 60 beats per minute. There is no forward diastolic flow or B wave. There is reverse flow in diastole (small arrows)

CHAPTER 4

Structural cardiac abnormalities – the venous atrial junction

In the complete morphological evaluation of a structural cardiac abnormality each connection within the heart should be sought. Once each connection is identified and recorded additional defects should be noted. It is important always to follow a logical sequence of analysis and not to be distracted by finding a defect in one cardiac segment. *All* the connections and possible additional lesions must be looked for, as combined defects will have quite a different prognosis from isolated anomalies. There are three connections to be considered on each side of the heart. These are the veno-atrial junction, the atrioventricular junction and the ventriculo-arterial junction.

The first step in the description of a cardiac abnormality is the identification of atrial situs. In some forms of complex congenital heart disease there has been an associated failure of correct lateralization in the early developing embryo. This produces two left sides in terms of thoracic or abdominal organs, or two right sides. Usually in left atrial isomerism there are also two morphological left atria, two left lungs and bronchi, multiple small spleens and a central liver. In right atrial isomerism, there are two morphological right atria, two right lungs and bronchi, a central liver and asplenia. Malrotation of the gut is common in both conditions. Both right and left atrial isomerism lead to abnormalities at the veno-atrial junction. In right isomerism, the pulmonary venous connection is abnormal. In left isomerism the systemic veins, usually the inferior vena cava, may drain abnormally.

Atrial situs is determined by examination of the aorta and inferior vena cava in the abdomen. Figure 1.30 shows the abdomen in cross-section. The aorta and inferior vena cava are seen lying in their normal relationship to the spine. The two vessels are positioned fairly symmetrically on either side of the vertebral body, with the aorta on the left, and the inferior vena cava slightly anterior and on the right. This should be checked by working out the fetal position. The aorta should lie on the same side of the fetus as the stomach and heart. The connection of the inferior vena cava to the right atrium should be noted. In left atrial isomerism the inferior vena cava is commonly interrupted and continues as the azygous vein behind the aorta. Only the aorta can be seen in the abdomen in Figure 4.1. This was a case of left atrial isomerism. In right atrial isomerism the abdominal vessels are both present but they tend to run together at one or other side of the abdomen (Figure 4.2). The pulmonary veins in this case drained behind the left-sided atrium to a common vein which then communicated directly with the right atrium (Figure 4.3). Figure 4.4 illustrates what has been described as the 'string' sign of right atrial isomerism. This represents a thin strand of atrial septum seen in the body of the combined atrial cavity.

Examination of the great vessels in the abdomen can be misleading in some rare circumstances. In one case we diagnosed atrial isomerism because the abdominal aorta and inferior vena cava lay on the right side of the spine closely related to each other. There was an atrioventricular septal defect and a double outlet right ventricle, the sort of combination of cardiac defects commonly associated with atrial isomerism. However, the fetus also had a diaphragmatic hernia with displacement of the heart into the right chest. At autopsy both abdominal vessels did indeed lie in the right abdomen, but this appears to have been due to the positional abnormality of the heart. There was normal atrial situs. Most cases of atrial isomerism are associated with complex congenital heart disease, although this is not an absolute rule. A common component of isomerism syndromes is an atrioventricular septal defect. When complete heart block occurs in association with structural heart disease, left atrial isomerism is nearly always present.

Abnormalities at the veno-atrial junction need not, however, always be related to atrial isomerism. Anomalies of pulmonary venous drainage most commonly occur as an isolated defect. The first clue to the diagnosis of total anomalous pulmonary venous drainage is the recognition of the rather non-specific sign of right to left ventricular disproportion. The right ventricle is dilated relative to the left. The pulmonary artery appears appreciably larger than the aorta. The left ventricular and aortic measurements are in the lower normal range for gestational age. There are three potential forms of total anomalous pulmonary venous drainage – supracardiac, cardiac and infracardiac. The only form which we have encountered prenatally to date has been the cardiac form. In this condition the pulmonary veins drain behind the left atrium to the coronary sinus which drains in turn to the right atrium (Figures 4.5, 4.6). Doppler estimation of blood flow can help this diagnosis. The ratio of R/L blood flow across either the atrio-ventricular or arterial valves is $>2:1$ as a consistent finding. At the same time the aortic blood flow is maintained at near normal levels. These findings can distinguish this cause of R/L ventricular disproportion from that seen in other conditions.

It seems likely that the other forms of total anomalous pulmonary venous drainage could be recognized. Pulmonary veins are nearly always identifiable draining to the left atrium in the normal heart. Absence of this finding in association with right ventricular dilatation should lead to a search for an ascending or descending common pulmonary vein. The unobstructed view of the posterior thorax in fetal life should allow such a collecting chamber to be more readily identified than is often possible postnatally.

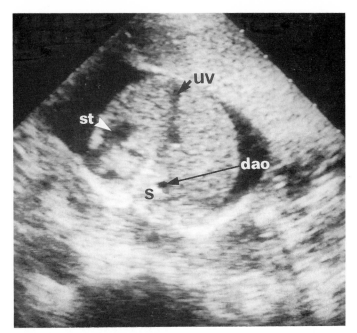

Figure 4.1 The abdomen is seen in cross-section at the level of the umbilical vein. The stomach can be seen in the left side of the abdomen. The aorta could be clearly seen pulsating in the moving image and lying almost directly anterior to the spine. The inferior vena cava could not be seen in this section. Nor could it be traced out of the right atrium in a long axis section of the fetus. This is left atrial isomerism

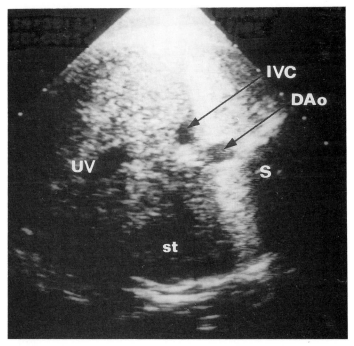

Figure 4.2 The abdomen is seen in cross-section. Both the inferior vena cava and the aorta lay to the right of the spine. This is right atrial isomerism

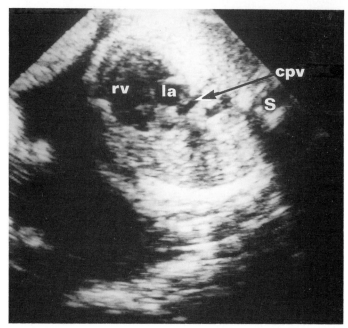

Figure 4.3 The left pulmonary veins are seen to drain into a common vein passing behind the left-sided atrium. This vein communicated directly with the right-sided atrium. This was associated with right atrial isomerism

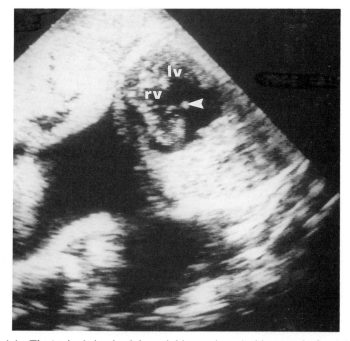

Figure 4.4 The 'string' sign in right atrial isomerism. A thin strand of atrial septum is seen within the atrial cavity. There is a common atrioventricular valve in this instance

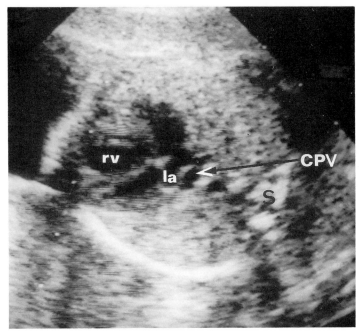

Figure 4.5 The right ventricle is dilated. There is seen to be a membrane which appears to be within or behind the left atrium. The pulmonary veins all drained to this chamber, which was a common pulmonary vein, lying behind the left atrium. It gave this appearance of the left atrium being divided. Slight posterior movement of the transducer allowed the connection of this vein to be seen in Figure 4.6

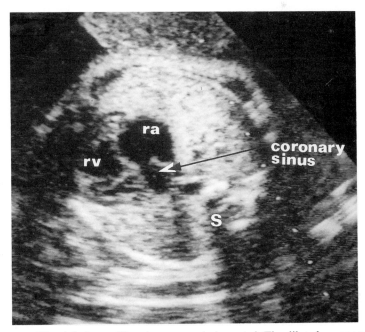

Figure 4.6 The right heart dilatation can again be noted. The dilated coronary sinus is seen draining to the right atrium. The common pulmonary vein seen in Figure 4.5 drained to this coronary sinus. The pulmonary venous return appeared unobstructed

CHAPTER 5

Structural cardiac abnormalities - the atrioventricular junction

The atrioventricular connection can show the following abnormalities: absence of left or right connection, common valve, double inlet, dysplastic or displaced connection. Rarely it may be appreciated that the atrioventricular connection is inverted, that is the right atrium connects to the morphological left ventricle, with the left atrium connected to a morphological right ventricle.

Absent left connection or mitral atresia occurs when there is no connection between the floor of the left atrium and the ventricular mass. The muscular tissue which separates the left atrium from the left ventricular cavity is continuous with the lateral wall of the ventricle (Figure 5.1). In earlier pregnancy the heart may have the appearance of a two- or three-chambered structure with the cavity or potential cavity of the left ventricle undetectable (Figures 5.2, 5.3). In Figure 5.2 there is a common atrium and one ventricular chamber, and in Figure 5.3 the atrial septum can be seen as a landmark pointing to where the crux of the heart can be seen. But in this case no left ventricle is found. In this orientation to the fetal chest with the heart positioned facing the transducer, failure to find four chambers must be a real and not a technical difficulty. Figure 5.4 shows an example of mitral atresia where the left ventricular cavity is seen but is much smaller than the right. The left ventricle has a small cavity in this case because of the presence of a ventricular septal defect. M-mode examination can sometimes be of help in the detection of a small ventricular cavity which cannot be seen on cross-sectional scanning. Figure 5.5 shows a small posterior ventricular chamber. The right ventricle in this case is appropriate for the gestational age; the left ventricle is very small for gestation. This is quite a different form of R/L ventricular disproportion than that described in the previous chapter where the right ventricle is dilated for the gestational age. Use of measurement charts can help to clarify the individual case. Doppler interrogation of the left atrioventricular valve in mitral atresia will fail to find forward flow through the mitral valve.

Absent right connection or tricuspid atresia occurs when there is no connection between the right atrium and right ventricle. This is illustrated in Figure 5.6 where a slit in the anterior myocardium represents the rudimentary right ventricle. The aorta in this case arises astride both the main left ventricular chamber and the rudimentary right ventricle. Figure 5.7 illustrates another case of tricuspid atresia: the image could be alternatively interpreted as of mitral atresia, but the main ventricle has no moderator band and appears smooth-walled in its apex, suggesting the morphology of a left ventricle. In addition, the atrioventricular valve attachment is only to the free wall of the ventricle, typical of a mitral valve. There was also an antero-superior rudimentary chamber. A rudimentary ventricle in this position is nearly always a right ventricle. A rudimentary left ventricle will be posterio-inferior in position.

In the normal heart the atrial and ventricular septa meet the two atrioventricular valves at the crux of the heart. This forms a cross at this point. However, this is normally a slightly offset cross as the tricuspid valve is inserted slightly more apically in the ventricular septum than the mitral. This is illustrated anatomically in Figure 5.8a and echocardiographically in Figure 5.8b.

An atrioventricular septal defect is a defect occurring at the crux of the heart. It may be partial when there is only an atrial defect, or complete where there are both atrial and ventricular components. A partial defect is illustrated in Figure 5.9. The crucial lower part of the atrial septum is absent and the normal offset appearance of differential valvular insertion is lost. The loss of differential insertion is often better seen when the ultrasound beam is projected directly up the ventricular septum as in positions 1 or 3 in Figure 1.5 (Figure 5.10). This defect used to be called an ostium primum atrial septal defect, although the term partial atrioventricular septal defect (AVSD) is now preferred. Care should be taken to confirm a partial atrioventricular septal defect from both positions 1 or 3 as well as seeing it in positions 2 or 4. This is because the appearance can sometimes be falsely produced in a normal heart if the four-chamber orientation is incorrect (Figure 5.11).

Figures 5.12a and 5.12b show an example of a complete atrioventricular septal defect in systole and diastole. The defect above and below the common atrioventricular valve can be seen. Again the normal characteristic appearance at the crux of the heart is lost, the valve forming a straight line bridging the defect when it is closed. Both partial and complete atrioventricular septal defects are commonly associated with Down's syndrome. The detection of this cardiac defect should therefore prompt a thorough search, firstly for other cardiac anomalies. The type of atrioventricular septal defect that occurs with atrial isomerism, and usually complex venous and arterial anomalies, will not be associated with Down's. On the other hand, if the defect is isolated to an AVSD with normal atrial situs other features of Down's should be sought by ultrasound, e.g. exomphalos, duodenal atresia, renal anomalies and basal neck pad of fat (Figure 5.13). Chromosome analysis should also be performed by amniocentesis or fetal blood sampling if indicated. The prognosis for successful operability in AVSDs can be influenced by dominance of one or other ventricle. Ventricular disproportion should therefore be noted if it is present. Figure 5.14 shows an example of a very small but complete atrioventricular defect where the right ventricle is considerably larger than the left.

If both atrioventricular valves drain predominantly to one ventricular chamber this is a double inlet connection. The mode of connection can be via two discrete atrioventricular valves or via a common valve. Our only examples of double inlet connection are of common valves (Figure 5.15). The common valve is directed mainly to the right ventricle, the left ventricular cavity being very small.

A defect not commonly seen in postnatal life is a dysplastic regurgitant tricuspid valve. However, this defect is frequently recognized as an isolated lesion prenatally. Figure 5.16 shows a four-chamber view in such a case. The tricuspid valve was not abnormally situated or inserted, but was lumpy and thickened on cross-sectional examination. The right ventricle and right atrium were both grossly dilated due to free tricuspid regurgitation as seen in Figure 5.17. There was no increased gradient across the tricuspid valve to suggest any degree of tricuspid stenosis. The cardiomegaly can be very gross (Figures 5.18a and 5.18b) and causes secondary lung hypoplasia by interfering with lung development in late pregnancy.

Another defect commonly recognized prenatally is Ebstein's anomaly. This is because it tends to lead to a regurgitant tricuspid valve and cardiomegaly. The cardiac enlargement is then noticed on a routine scan. The septal leaflet of the tricuspid valve is displaced into the right ventricle in this anomaly. Various degrees of displacement are possible. Figure 5.19 shows the tricuspid valve inserted near the apex; Figure 5.20 shows tethering of the valve to the septum with the functional valve orifice in the mid-cavity of the right ventricle. Figure 5.21 shows an early example of a mild form of Ebstein's anomaly where the difference of displacement from normal was difficult to appreciate. This valve was not regurgitant and there was no cardiomegaly.

Congenitally corrected transposition occurs when the left atrium connects to the morphological right ventricle which then gives rise to the aorta: the right atrium is connected to the morphological left ventricle which gives rise to the pulmonary artery (Figure 5.22). Ebstein's anomaly is a commonly associated feature of this condition occurring in the left-sided atrioventricular valve, the tricuspid valve. This was present in this example.

Thus all possible abnormalities at the crux of the heart can be recognised prenatally. Abnormalities of atrioventricular connection can be accurately analysed if evaluation is approached systematically.

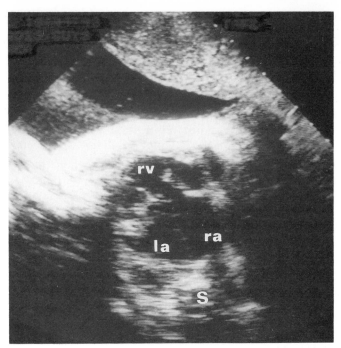

Figure 5.1 The floor of the left atrium is formed of thick muscular tissue which is continuous with the left ventricular wall. There is no direct communication between the left atrium and the ventricular mass. This is mitral atresia

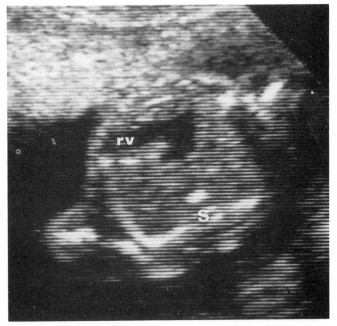

Figure 5.2 The thorax is sectioned to show a four-chamber view but only two cavities can be seen, a large common atrium and a right ventricular chamber. No left ventricular cavity can be distinguished within the ventricular mass

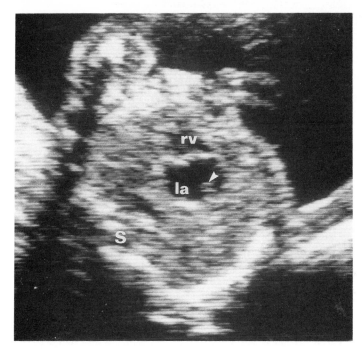

Figure 5.3 Again the thorax is sectioned to image four chambers, but only the right ventricle is seen. The atrial septum (arrow) is pointing to the crux of the heart but no left-sided ventricular chamber is seen. In both Figures 5.3 and 5.4 the fetal heart is facing the transducer and the beam is correctly orientated square across the chest. Failure to find four chambers in this view must be a real rather than a technical difficulty

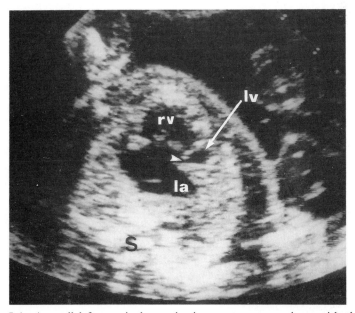

Figure 5.4 A small left ventricular cavity is seen to communicate with the right ventricle through a ventricular septal defect (arrow). There is again no direct left atrial communication to the ventricular mass

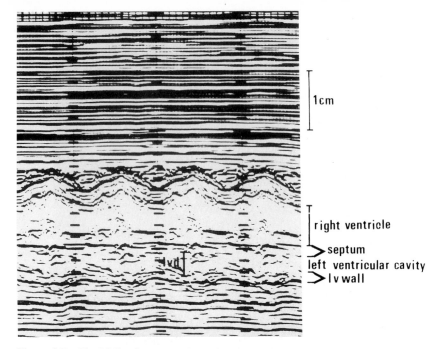

1cm

right ventricle
septum
left ventricular cavity
lv wall

Figure 5.5 The M-line is swept across the right ventricle seen on the cross-sectional image in Figure 5.3. The M-mode echocardiogram displays the presence of a small posterior left ventricular chamber which was not detectable on cross-sectional scanning. Measurement of this chamber and comparison with the graph of normal left ventricular dimensions (Figure 2.6) shows that this left ventricle is very small for the gestational age

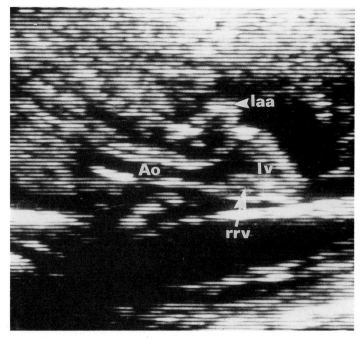

Figure 5.6 The aorta is seen arising astride a ventricular septal defect. A slit in the anterior myocardium represents the rudimentary right ventricle. No communication was found between the right atrium and the right ventricle

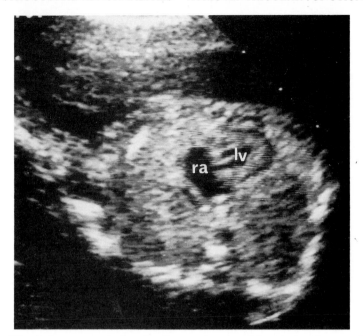

Figure 5.7   Only one ventricular chamber can be seen although the ultrasound beam is positioned correctly to image four chambers. The one ventricle seen had no coarse trabeculation in its apex. The attachment of the atrioventricular valve was all to the free wall of the ventricle with none to the septal surface. This is characteristic of a mitral valve. This therefore is a left ventricle. There was a discordant atrioventricular connection

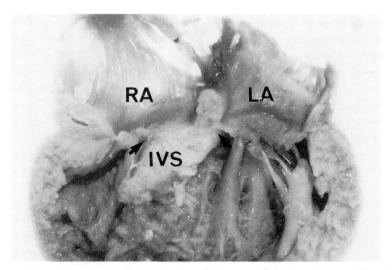

Figure 5.8a   A close-up anatomical view of the crux of the heart is seen. The mitral valve can be seen to be inserted slightly higher in the septum than the tricuspid valve. the arrows indicate the points of insertion of each valve

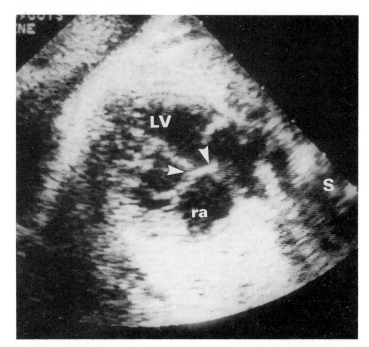

Figure 5.8b The offset cross appearance at the crux of the heart can be seen. The atrial and ventricular septa and the two atrioventricular valves meet at the crux but the tricuspid valve is slightly below the junction of the other three

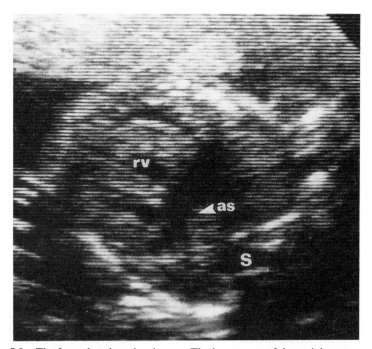

Figure 5.9 The four-chamber view is seen. The lower part of the atrial septum which should meet the ventricular septum at the crux is absent. The atrioventricular valves insert at the same point in the ventricular septum i.e. the normal offset appearance is lost

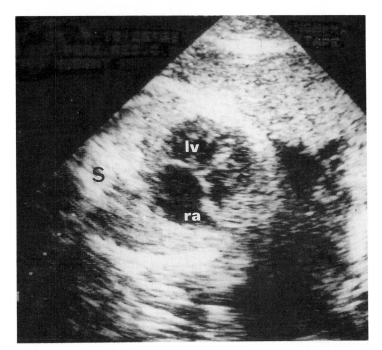

Figure 5.10 The crux of the heart is imaged almost from the apex. This allows the simultaneous insertion of the atrioventricular valves, characteristic of an atrioventricular septal defect, to be seen clearly

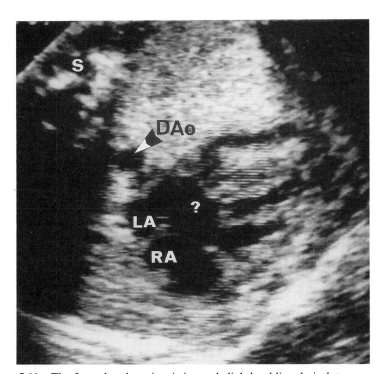

Figure 5.11 The four-chamber view is imaged slightly obliquely in late pregnancy. This can give an artificial appearance of a defect of the primum part of the atrial septum. To confirm such a 'defect' it is necessary to image it also from the apex. In this case this possible 'defect' was not confirmed in this view

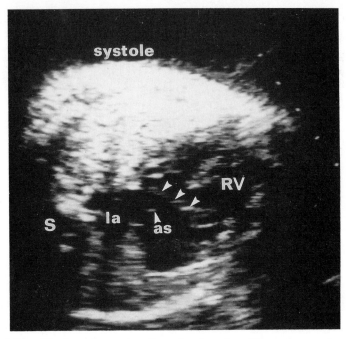

Figure 5.12a The heart is seen in a four-chamber view. The common valve (arrows) is seen closed, bridging an atrial and ventricular defect

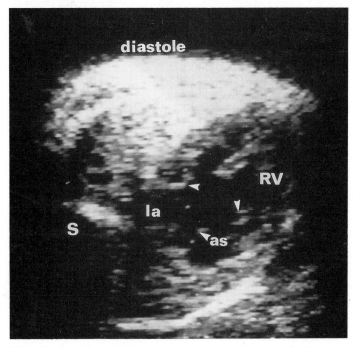

Figure 5.12b In diastole when the common atrioventricular valve is open (arrows) there is a large defect seen at the crux of the heart

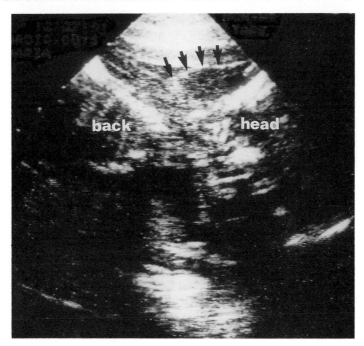

Figure 5.13 There appears to be a fatty lump of tissue at the base of the skull behind the neck. This arouses suspicion of Down's syndrome

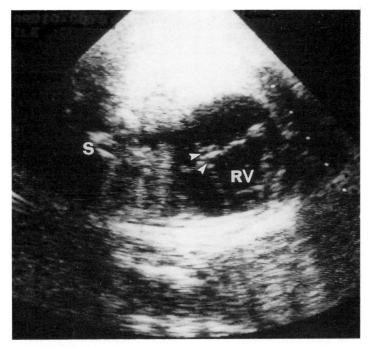

Figure 5.14 There are very small atrial and ventricular components to this complete atrioventricular septal defect. The right ventricle is nearly twice the left ventricle in size. This degree of right ventricular dominance may influence the surgical result

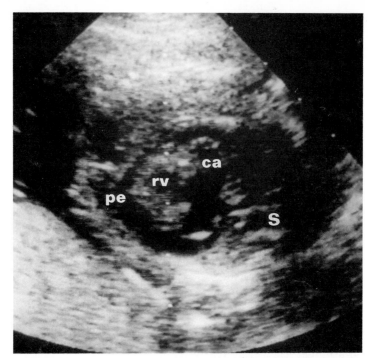

Figure 5.15 There is a complete atrioventricular septal defect but the valve is directed towards the right ventricle. The left ventricle was very small. There is also a pericardial effusion seen in this patient

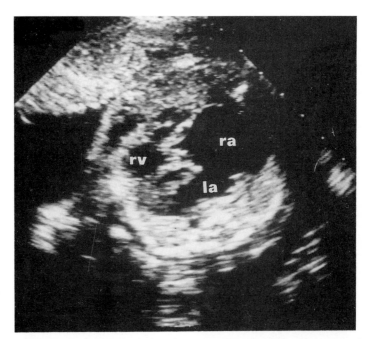

Figure 5.16 The heart is seen in the four-chamber view. The heart occupies over half the thorax. The right atrium and right ventricle are grossly dilated. Although dysplastic in appearance the tricuspid valve was not displaced. There appears to be an atrial septal defect in addition

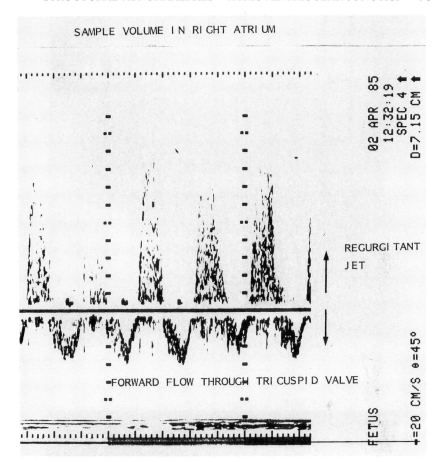

Figure 5.17   With the sample volume in the right atrium, forward flow through the tricuspid valve can be seen with gross regurgitation in systole

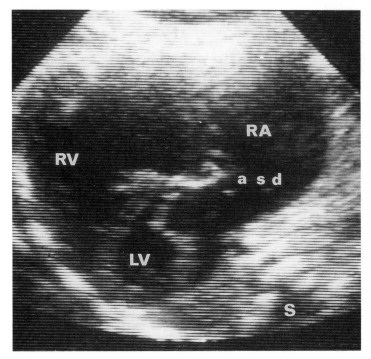

Figure 5.18a   The cardiac enlargement in this case of tricuspid dysplasia was very gross. This causes lung compression and thus lung hypoplasia

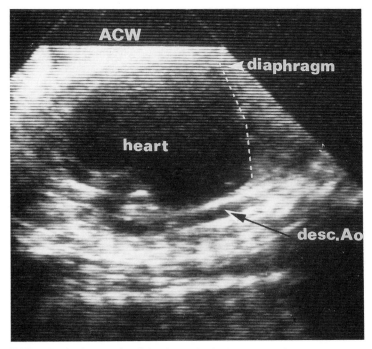

Figure 5.18b   In the long axis of the fetus the heart appeared to occupy nearly the whole thorax

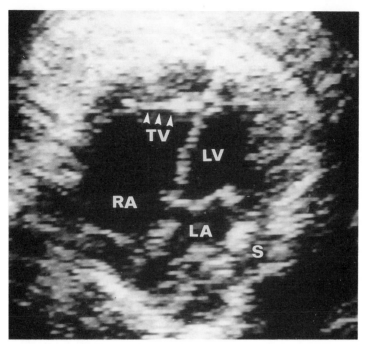

Figure 5.19   The heart fills nearly the whole thorax in a four-chamber view. The right atrium is greatly enlarged with the tricuspid valve (arrows) displaced into the apex of the right ventricle

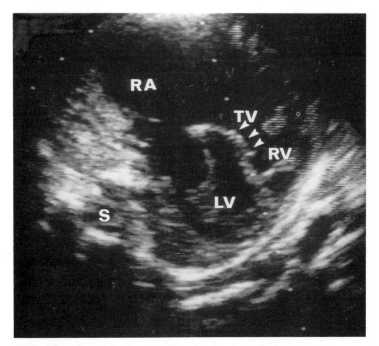

Figure 5.20   The tricuspid valve is tethered to the ventricular septum (arrows). The functional orifice of the valve was in the mid-cavity of the right ventricle. The right atrium is grossly dilated and the tricuspid valve was freely regurgitant

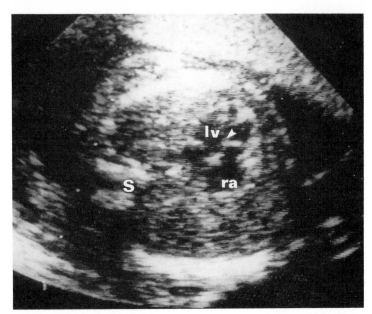

Figure 5.21 The normal differential insertion of the tricuspid valve appears exaggerated in this example. This is because there was Ebstein's anomaly of the tricuspid valve with slight apical displacement of the septal attachment of the valve (arrow)

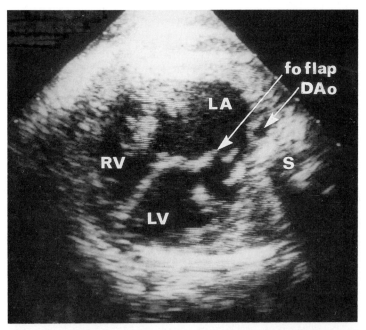

Figure 5.22 The heart lies with the apex pointing to the right. The left-sided atrium is the left atrium. It could be identified as such by the presence within it of the foramen ovale flap and the insertion of the pulmonary veins (not seen in this section). The left atrium also lay on the descending aorta. However, the left atrium was connected, via a displaced tricuspid valve, to the right ventricle. This could be distinguished from its trabecular morphology. In other projections it could be seen that the right ventricle gave rise to the aorta, the left ventricle to the pulmonary artery. Thus, this was atrioventricular and ventriculoarterial discordance or corrected transposition

CHAPTER 6

Structural cardiac abnormalities – the ventriculo-arterial junction

Normally two great arteries arise from the heart, the aorta from the left ventricle, and the pulmonary artery from the right ventricle. The two great arteries cross each other at right angles at their origin (Figures 6.1a, b). The great arteries are of similar size but the pulmonary artery is slightly larger than the aorta in cross-sectional diameter. The abnormalities that can be seen at the ventriculo-arterial junction include atresia or stenosis of one or other great artery, aortic override or inappropriate connection, i.e. transposition or double outlet.

Aortic atresia is commonly associated with mitral atresia to make up the hypoplastic left heart syndrome. There is no forward flow into the left ventricle. The aorta fills retrogradely from the ductus arteriosus. An example of this condition is seen in Figure 6.2a. The left ventricle is a small solid chamber. The ascending aorta is very small in relationship to the pulmonary artery (Figure 6.2b). In one pregnancy seen in late gestation a very narrow aortic arch was seen in comparison to the ductus (Figures 6.3, 6.4). The Doppler sample probe could only find retrograde flow in the arch, coming from the pulmonary artery (Figure 6.5). This is aortic atresia.

Pulmonary atresia is where no patent connection is present between the right ventricle and the pulmonary artery. This can take a variety of forms. The form most commonly seen postnatally is where the right ventricle is a small hypertrophied chamber and there is no visible outflow tract. The pulmonary arteries are usually small and may not be confluent. Figure 6.6a shows a four-chamber view where the right ventricle is seen to be small and thick-walled. Figure 6.6b, from the same patient shows that there are confluent pulmonary arteries although the small main pulmonary artery ends blindly quite a distance from the right ventricle. Figure 6.7 shows a similar fetus at 18 weeks gestation, where the right ventricle is hypoplastic. No main pulmonary artery was found arising from the heart. The right pulmonary artery underneath the arch was extremely small.

A much more common form of pulmonary atresia seen prenatally is found in association with tricuspid regurgitation. This can occur in the setting of tricuspid dysplasia or Ebstein's anomaly. There is no forward flow through the pulmonary artery although the site of connection can usually be well seen. There is usually a thickened membrane seen occluding the pulmonary outflow at the valve site (Figure 6.8). It is possible that this form of pulmonary atresia is a secondary phenomenon, i.e. the pulmonary valve cusps become adherent as a result of the inability of the right ventricle to overcome pulmonary artery pressure. When the right ventricle contracts the blood leaks back through the tricuspid valve. Frequently the pulmonary artery is a good size (Figure 6.9). However, the cardiac dilatation as a result of the tricuspid incompetence impairs lung development and leads to a poor prognosis. This form of pulmonary atresia with a dilated right ventricle is rarely seen postnatally but is by far the more frequent form seen prenatally. This is because the cardiac dilatation is readily detected prenatally and also because there is a high incidence of immediate postnatal loss.

Stenosis of the aortic or pulmonary valve is usually recognized by a disparity in their relative sizes, the stenosed vessel being disproportionately small. This is seen in Figure 6.10, where the aorta is very tiny. Only a pinhole orifice was found at postmortem. There was associated endocardial fibroelastosis of the left ventricle and left atrium. The dilatation of both cavities can be seen (Figure 6.10).

Less commonly, thickening of the arterial valve or post-stenotic dilatation can be seen. Figure 6.11 shows some thickening of the pulmonary valve. There was an increased velocity of flow to $2\,\mathrm{m\,s^{-1}}$ across it, implying a gradient of about 16 mmHg. These findings were confirmed postnatally.

In the long axis view of the left ventricle the normal feature of aortic septal continuity can be appreciated. Loss of this feature produces aortic override. Care should be exercised in interpreting this finding as a misleading appearance can be produced. This is seen in Figure 6.12 where the ultrasound beam is incorrectly positioned producing a false impression of aortic override. True aortic override can, however, be seen (Figures 6.13, 6.14). When the aorta is definitely overriding, the pulmonary artery must be sought. If the pulmonary artery arises from the right ventricle the diagnosis must be tetralogy of Fallot; if it arises from the aorta it is truncus arteriosus; if the pulmonary artery does not connect to the heart the diagnosis is pulmonary atresia with ventricular septal defect. Figure 6.15b shows the pulmonary artery arising from the back of the single arterial trunk seen in Figure 6.15a. This is therefore an example of truncus arteriosus. The infundibular stenosis of tetralogy of Fallot may not be developed prenatally and the pulmonary outflow tract may appear widely patent (Figure 6.16). This appearance can change throughout pregnancy. We have observed a normally proportioned size of pulmonary artery in early pregnancy changing to a relatively small pulmonary artery as pregnancy progressed. Thus a favourable appearance for corrective surgery became unfavourable.

Transposition of the great arteries can also be recognized prenatally. The normal features of the great arteries crossing over each other will be lost. The great vessels arise in parallel orientation (Figure 6.17). The two arterial valves are at the same level in transposition rather than the normal situation of the pulmonary artery anterior and cranial to the aorta. The great artery that arises from the right ventricle can be seen to give rise to the arch and head and neck vessels. This arch will appear much more 'open' than the normal appearance of the tight hook of the arch (Figure 6.18). The great artery arising in the centre of the chest can be seen to branch into the right and left pulmonary arteries (Figure 6.19a). Figure 6.19b from the same patient shows the aorta anterior and lateral to the pulmonary artery, and slightly above it.

In double outlet connection the two great arteries can both be seen to arise anterior to the ventricular septum (Figure 6.20). The posterior great artery can be seen to be the pulmonary artery by following it to its branches. It is slightly smaller than the aorta suggesting a degree of pulmonary stenosis. In the case illustrated in Figure 6.21 the arch could be seen arising from the right ventricle. The main pulmonary artery also arose from this ventricle, but it was extremely small and the valve atretic. This, therefore, was double outlet right ventricle with pulmonary atresia. Figure 6.22 shows another example of double outlet right ventricle where the heart was imaged in a different projection to show the aorta arising anterior to the ventricular septum. The pulmonary artery also could be found arising anterior to the septum in this case.

The unobstructed views, in fetal life, of the heart and the relationships of the great vessels are greatly to the advantage of prenatal cardiac study. If the ventriculo-arterial connection on each side of the heart is logically and sequentially followed, abnormalities can be identified and confirmed in a variety of projections. Even though these projections may not be those familiar from postnatal echocardiography, the continuous sweep of the prenatal scan can allow accurate identification of each structure.

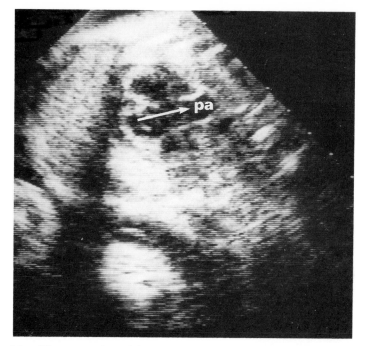

Figure 6.1a The connection of the pulmonary outflow tract to the main pulmonary artery runs across our picture from left to right in the direction of the arrow

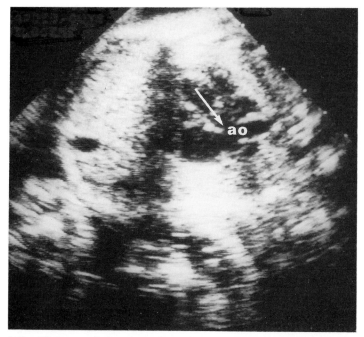

Figure 6.1b Slight angulation down from the section seen in Figure 6.1a allows the left ventricular-aortic root connection to be seen. Note that the direction of this connection (arrow) is almost at right angles to that between the right ventricle and pulmonary artery

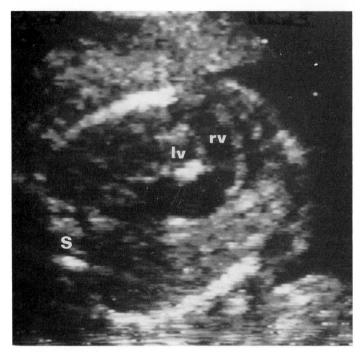

Figure 6.2a The heart is seen in the four-chamber projection. The left ventricle appears as a solid echogenic mass of tissue with a minute cavity

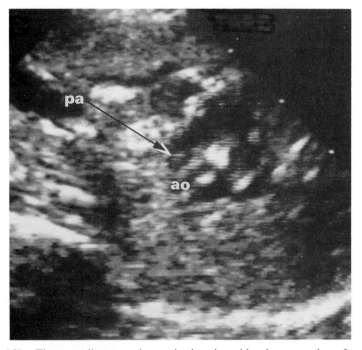

Figure 6.2b The ascending aorta is seen in the tricuspid pulmonary plane. It can be seen to be less than half the diameter of the pulmonary artery in size. No forward flow through the aortic valve could be detected in the aortic root by Doppler examination

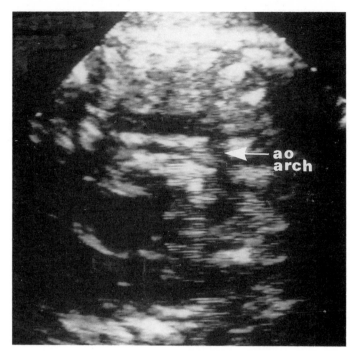

Figure 6.3 The aortic arch appeared narrow compared to the descending aorta and pulmonary artery ductal connection seen in Figure 6.4

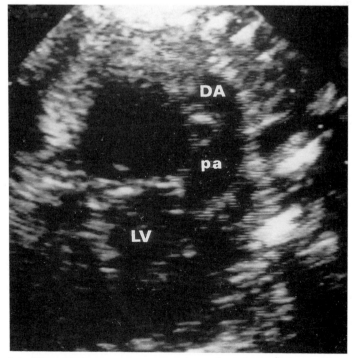

Figure 6.4 The pulmonary artery arose from the left ventricle in this case. The ductus arteriosus was larger than the aortic arch in internal dimension

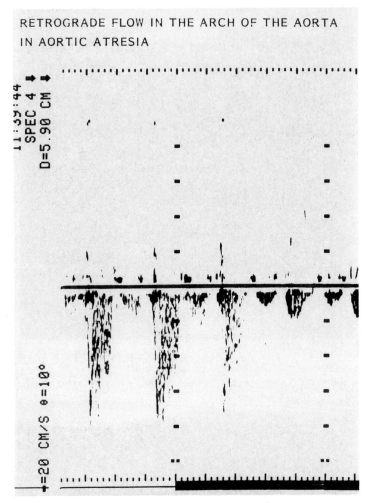

Figure 6.5 Positioning the Doppler sample volume in the arch of the aorta, only retrograde flow could be recorded. Thus the arch of the aorta was being perfused entirely from the ductus arteriosus

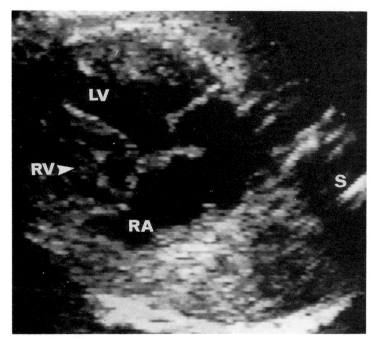

Figure 6.6a The cavity of the right ventricle was nearly completely obscured by the hypertrophied walls. The tricuspid valve ring was small with limited excursion of the valve cusps

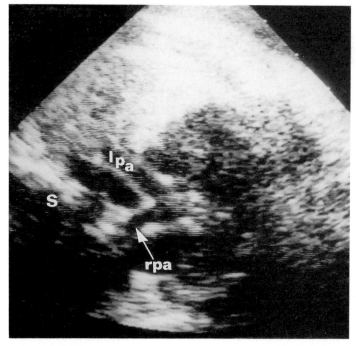

Figure 6.6b Confluent left and right pulmonary arteries could be found on searching the upper thorax. However, the main pulmonary artery ended blindly some distance from the right ventricle

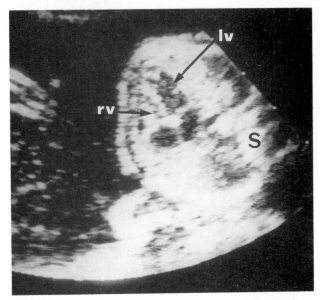

Figure 6.7   In an 18 week fetus the right ventricle could be seen to be much smaller and thicker than the left. No main pulmonary artery could be found arising from the right heart. This is pulmonary atresia

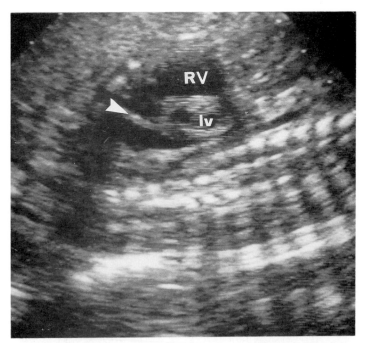

Figure 6.8   The heart is seen in the short axis of the left ventricle. The right ventricle can be seen in this view to be dilated. There is a dense membrane occluding the right ventricular outflow tract where the pulmonary valve is normally seen (arrow). The Doppler sample volume positioned beyond this membrane could not detect forward flow in the pulmonary artery

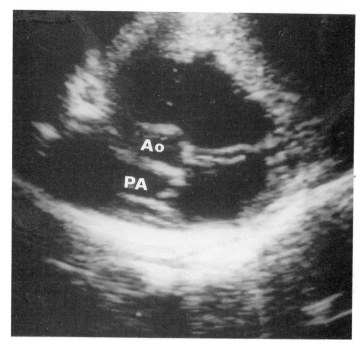

Figure 6.9 The aorta is seen in the centre of the heart. The pulmonary outflow tract and main pulmonary artery 'wrap' around anterior to the aorta. The main pulmonary artery is a normal size in proportion to the aorta. However, in fetal life there was no forward flow through this pulmonary valve

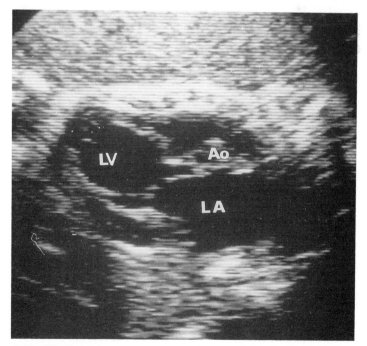

Figure 6.10 The heart is seen in the long axis of the left ventricle. The left atrium and ventricle are dilated. They were also poorly contracting. The aorta is very small particularly at its origin. This was critical aortic stenosis with endocardial fibroelastosis

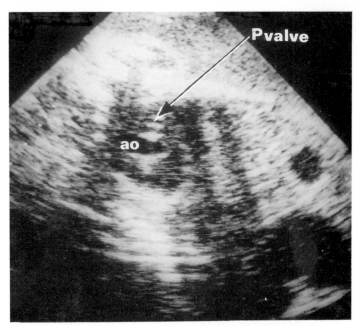

Figure 6.11 The heart is seen in the tricuspid pulmonary plane. In the moving image the pulmonary valve could be seen to be much thicker than the aortic valve and somewhat dysplastic. There was a small gradient, detected on Doppler evaluation, across the pulmonary valve

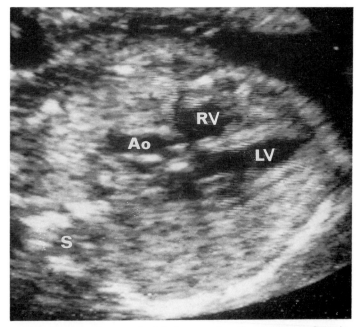

Figure 6.12 Care must be exercised in interpreting the suspicion of aortic override. In a high long axis view of the left ventricle a false impression of aortic override, as in this picture, can be seen. If the long axis is lined up so that the posterior wall of the aorta is continuous with the anterior cusp of the mitral valve, the septum should be continuous with the anterior wall of the aorta in the normal heart

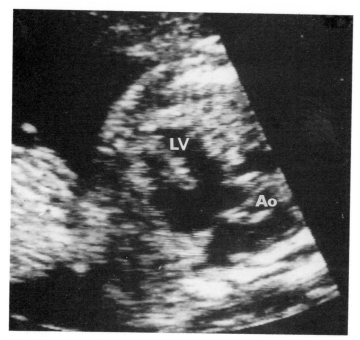

Figure 6.13 The aorta arises astride a large ventricular septal defect. In no section of the heart could the anterior wall of the aorta be connected to the ventricular septum

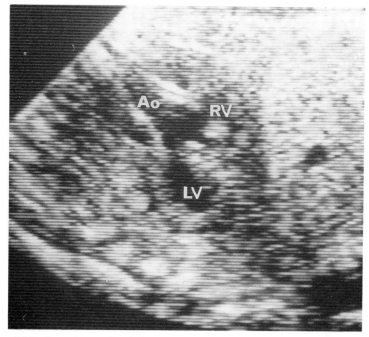

Figure 6.14 In a short axis of the left ventricle section, aortic override can also be identified. The aorta is seen arising astride a large ventricular septal defect

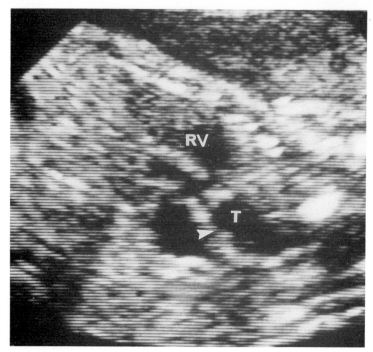

Figure 6.15a Only one arterial trunk could be found arising from the ventricular mass. This great artery overrode the crest of the ventricular septum. Scanning across the trunk revealed the main pulmonary artery arising from the posterior aspect of the common trunk in the position of the arrow. This is seen in Figure 6.15b

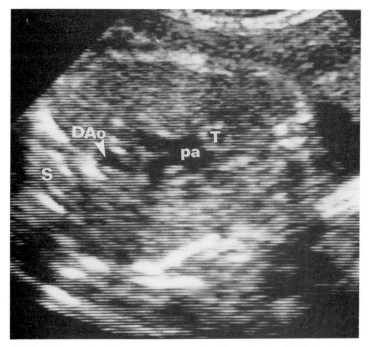

Figure 6.15b The main pulmonary artery arises from the back of the single arterial trunk. Branching of the main pulmonary artery into right and left pulmonary arteries can be seen

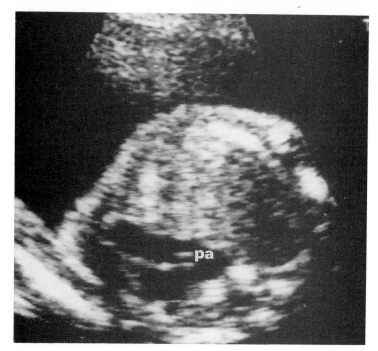

Figure 6.16 The main pulmonary artery and right ventricular outflow tract is seen. There is no visible narrowing of either structure. This was a case of tetralogy of Fallot seen in early pregnancy. Significant infundibular stenosis had not yet developed although the anterior displacement of the infundibular septum and typical ventricular septal defect were present

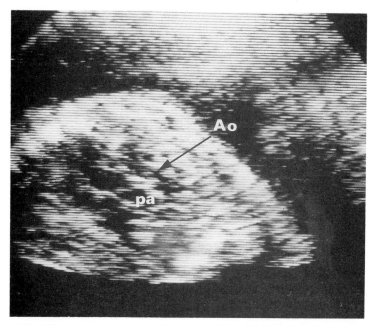

Figure 6.17 The two great arteries arise in parallel orientation. The two valve rings are seen side by side. The connection of each great artery from the ventricles to the descending aorta must be followed to make an accurate diagnosis when this sign is recognized

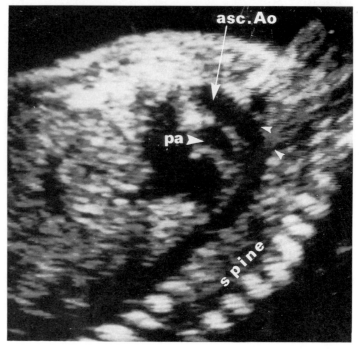

Figure 6.18   The two great arteries arise in parallel orientation. However, the anterior great artery gives rise to the arch of the aorta with head and neck vessels (arrows). This is the aorta, yet it arises close to the chest wall and the arch is a much wider curve than normal (see Figure 1.19b). Scanning in other planes showed the aorta to be connected to the right ventricle and the pulmonary artery to the left ventricle. This therefore is transposition of the great arteries

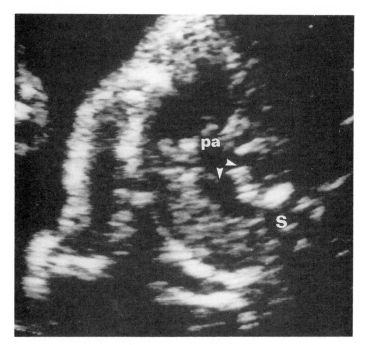

Figure 6.19a The great artery which branched into left and right pulmonary arteries (arrows) arose in the centre of the chest

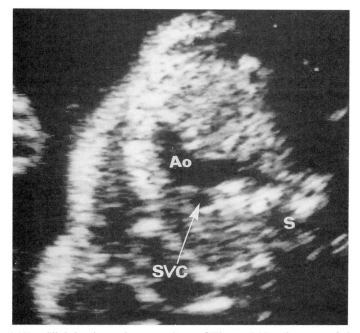

Figure 6.19b Slightly above the scan plane of Figure 6.19a, the crest of the aortic arch could be seen arising anterior, lateral and to the right of the central pulmonary artery

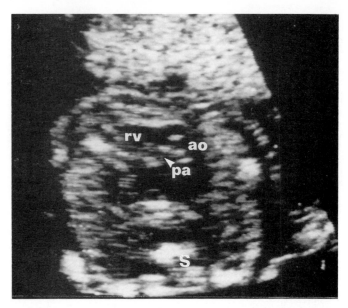

Figure 6.20   Both great arteries can be seen arising from the right ventricle. Both are anterior to the ventricular septum. By following both great arteries to their connection to the descending aorta it could be seen that the anterior larger great artery was the aorta, and the posterior great artery the pulmonary artery. The size disparity between the two suggests a degree of pulmonary stenosis

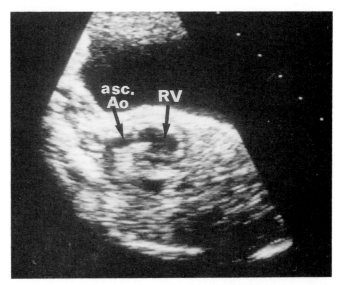

Figure 6.21   The ascending aorta is seen giving rise to the arch. It arises close to the anterior chest wall from the right ventricle. An atretic pulmonary artery could be visualized beneath the aorta

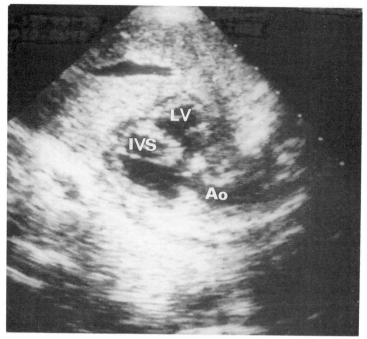

Figure 6.22 A short axis view of the left ventricle where the aorta could be seen to arise anterior to the ventricular septum. The pulmonary artery also arose from the right ventricle. Thus this was double outlet right ventricle

CHAPTER 7

Structural cardiac abnormalities – the aortic arch

Anomalies of the aortic arch can be detected in prenatal life. The first clue to an aortic arch anomaly is usually the recognition of a disparity between RV and LV size and PA to aortic root size. The right ventricle is slightly greater than normal size with the left ventricle slightly smaller (Figures 7.1a, b and c). The pulmonary artery is dilated relative to the aorta (Figures 7.2a, b and c). Doppler evaluation of blood flow will show a ratio of TV/MV of greater than 2:1 (normal range) 0.8–1.8 and absolute aortic flow is below the normal range. The more severe the aortic arch lesion, the more abnormal the blood flow results. Figure 7.3 shows the normal range of aortic blood flow throughout pregnancy with two cases of aortic arch anomaly plotted. The case with severe arch hypoplasia had a much smaller blood flow than the case with coarctation and relatively mild isthmal hypoplasia.

Figures 7.4 and 7.5 illustrate examples of an interrupted aorta. The small ascending aorta branches into head and neck vessels and does not form an aortic arch. Great care should be exercised in interpreting the failure to find an aortic arch, however. The arch can be difficult to visualize in every case: its position can be distorted if pleural effusions are present or if intrathoracic organs are displaced. Also the arch will not be readily visualized in a fetus with a right-sided arch. Transverse views taken of the upper thorax in order to image the aortic arch in the neck should be carefully studied in cases where the longitudinal views of the arch are difficult to find. Only when positive identification of the unusual branching end of the ascending aorta has been made should interrupted arch be diagnosed. The small absolute size of the aorta in this condition and the commonly associated ventricular septal defect would be important additional clues in this diagnosis.

Coarctation of the aorta can only be inferred from the non-specific features of RV > LV and PA > Ao where the aortic arch is complete. A discrete coarctation membrane cannot be discerned on direct examination of the arch itself in early pregnancy. This is perhaps because the plane of the membrane is parallel to the ultrasound beam in the aortic arch view and may be below the resolution of the imaging equipment. This theory is illustrated in Figure 7.6.

In our experience in the last six years we have found certain groups of mothers to be at higher risk of having a child with coarctation than others. These include mothers with coarctation themselves or in the father and those mothers who have had a previous child with a left-sided obstructive lesion; hypoplastic left heart syndrome, mitral or aortic stenosis, atresia or coarctation. An affected parent may have up to a 1-in-10 risk of recurrence[27]: a previous child with a left-sided lesion may indicate a risk of 1-in-15 to approximately 1-in-30[19], a little higher than the 1-in-50 commonly quoted risk. In every patient, of course, R/L ventricular and arterial size should be consciously checked but in these high risk patients this should be given careful attention and Doppler estimation of flow through all four cardiac valves included in the study. Coarctation can also coexist with extracardiac anomalies, characteristically with cystic hygroma (Figure 7.7). Turner's syndrome was the underlying cause of cystic hygroma, non-immune hydrops and coarctation in this case.

We have now observed in several cases a changing appearance of coarctation during intrauterine life. In early pregnancy the diagnosis of coarctation has been inferred from R/L disproportional flow characteristics but the appearance of the arch has been favourable for surgery, i.e. the distal arch and isthmal region have been a normal size in proportion to the rest of the aorta. However, by the end of pregnancy in some cases the arch and isthmus began to look very small in relation to the growth of other structures and much less favourable for corrective surgery. Figure 7.8a shows the arch in the neck compared to the duct in a normal patient. Figure 7.8b shows a good sized arch which narrowed at the isthmus before a coarctation. Figure 7.8c shows more severe arch and isthmal hypoplasia also occurring with coarctation. We have seen two cases (Figure 7.3), starting at 18 weeks, with similar appearance and flow characteristics where the absolute flow in the aorta became much less in one case than the other as pregnancy progressed. This was associated with a much greater severity of arch hypoplasia at term in the fetus with lower aortic flow. Thus coarctation can be detected in early pregnancy but it can be extremely difficult to give an accurate prognosis based on the appearance of the arch at this stage.

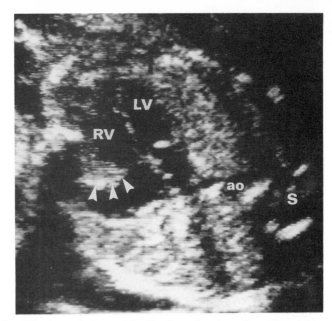

Figure 7.1a The heart is imaged in the four-chamber view. The right ventricle is slightly dilated relative to the left. The mass of tissue in the region of the insertion of the tricuspid valve into the right ventricular wall (arrows) is a common appearance in association with right ventricular dilatation, from any cause. It does not imply abnormality of tricuspid valve or right ventricle but simply means that the right ventricle is dilated

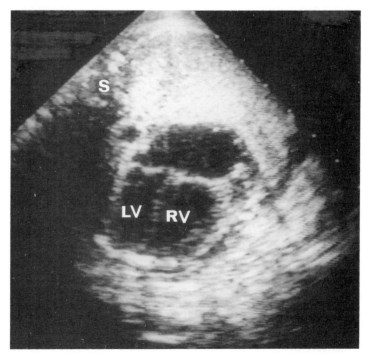

Figure 7.1b Another example of the ventricular disproportion that occurs in coarctation of the aorta. In this case the difference is quite subtle. The thickened region of tricuspid valve insertion is again seen but it is less conspicuous than in Figure 7.1a

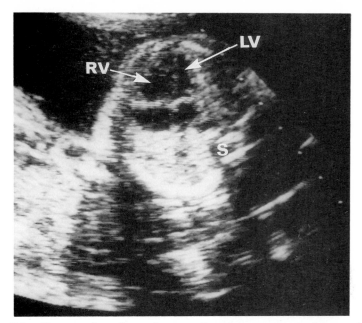

Figure 7.1c One complete rib can be seen, thus the operator can be sure that the horizontal section is correct. Yet the two ventricles appear distinctly different in size. This arouses strong suspicion of coarctation of the aorta in the non-hydropic fetus and where the pulmonary veins are seen to connect normally as here. Right ventricular dilatation in the context of fetal hydrops may have other haemodynamic implications

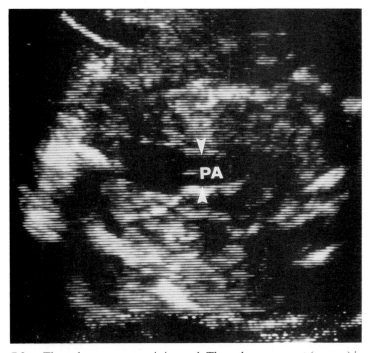

Figure 7.2a The pulmonary artery is imaged. The pulmonary root (arrows) is nearly twice the size of the aorta which lies immediately below it in Figure 7.2b. The pulmonary artery is normally only slightly larger than the aorta in size

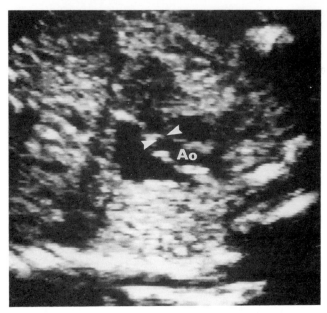

Figure 7.2b   The aorta is imaged at the same magnification just below the pulmonary artery seen in Figure 7.2a. It is appreciably smaller (arrows) than the pulmonary artery

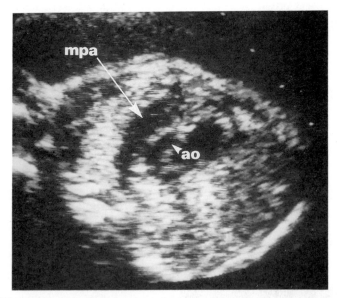

Figure 7.2c   The origin of the aorta and main pulmonary artery are compared here in the same section in a further example of a case of coarctation. The main pulmonary artery is about twice the dimension of the ascending aorta

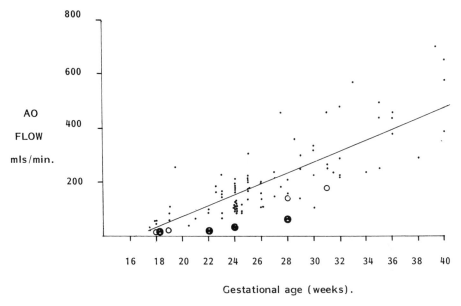

Figure 7.3   The calculated aortic blood flow throughout pregnancy is plotted. The circles indicate cases of coarctation of the aorta. The case with severe arch hypoplasia (closed circles) has lower blood flow than the one with mild isthmal hypoplasia (open circles) with advancing gestation

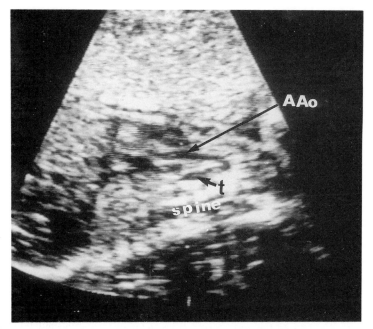

Figure 7.4   Only a tiny ascending aorta could be found. It branched into two head and neck vessels in the inlet of the thorax, where the aorta lay on the trachea. The trachea is often seen as a fluid-filled tube which can be seen extending from the neck to the mid-thorax

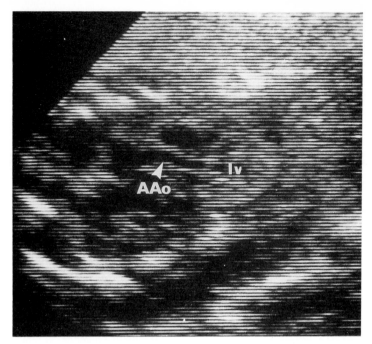

Figure 7.5 A very narrow aorta arises from the left ventricle. It widens and branches at the top of the thorax

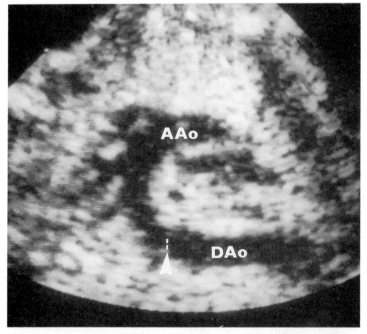

Figure 7.6 The arch of the aorta is seen from the usual projection in prenatal life. The site where infantile coarctation would be is marked. This would be a thin membrane projecting into the lumen of the aorta. In this projection this membrane would be parallel to the ultrasound beam and below the resolution capability of the machine certainly in early pregnancy. Therefore a normal appearance of this part of the aorta does not exclude a discrete coarctation

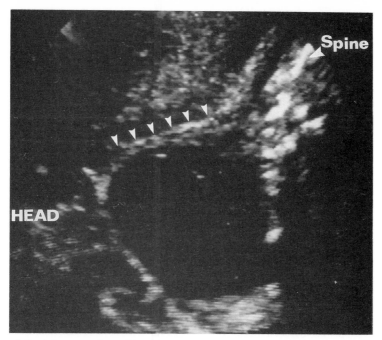

Figure 7.7 A large cystic swelling is seen in the region of the neck. It can be loculated. This is typical of cystic hygroma. Approximately half the affected fetuses will have Turner's syndrome. Coarctation of the aorta is a well-recognised association with Turner's syndrome

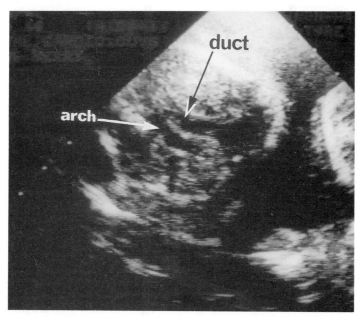

Figure 7.8a Examination of the inlet of the thorax in transverse section in the normal fetus should show the arch and the duct of similar size and even calibre meeting in front of the spine

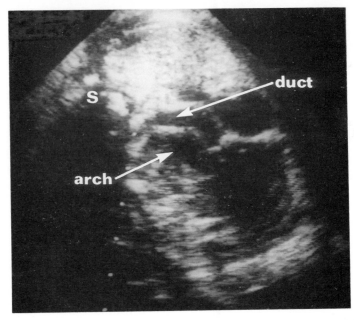

Figure 7.8b   The duct and arch are seen to meet anterior to the spine but the arch appears to become narrower just before the junction in the region of the isthmus

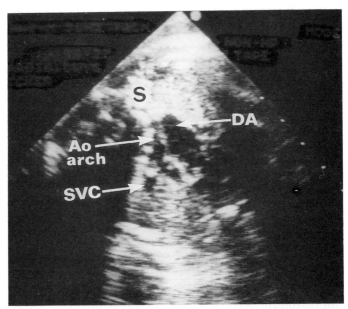

Figure 7.8c   The duct can be seen to be much wider than the arch and isthmus which are very narrow in this patient

CHAPTER 8

Structural cardiac abnormalities – additional defects

During the examination of the cardiac connections and aortic arch, additional defects will frequently be noticed. However, after the connections are established a conscious search for additional defects should be made.

The sort of moderate size secundum atrial septal defect that presents in childhood will not be distinguishable, in normal circumstances, from the foramen ovale, which can always be seen. It would be possible to establish a normal size range for the foramen ovale throughout pregnancy, but to us this seems an unnecessarily elaborate technique for diagnosing a defect that will not affect a child's wellbeing or life expectancy. We therefore accept that small to moderate secundum atrial septal defects are outside the confidence limits of the routine fetal echocardiogram. Large secundum defects are detectable however in the setting of gross atrioventricular valve incompetence (see Figure 5.16), or a common atrium. Figure 8.1 illustrates an unusual case where the only atrial septum to be seen was a stub of primum tissue at the insertion of the two atrioventricular valves. In this fetus there was in addition a small trabecular ventricular septal defect (Figure 8.2). There was also complete heart block and left atrial isomerism. Although this combination was more likely to be associated with an atrioventricular septal defect, a clear rim of tissue above and below two discrete atrioventricular valve orifices was clearly seen. The diagnosis of large secundum atrial septal defect and trabecular ventricular septal defect in the setting of atrial isomerism was confirmed at autopsy. The case emphasizes the importance of describing accurately what is seen (or not seen) on the fetal echocardiogram. The study should not be interpreted to fit with preconceived ideas derived from knowledge of postnatal paediatric cardiology or echocardiography.

Unusual and unlikely combinations of defects are not uncommonly seen prenatally. The reason many of these unusual defects are not seen postnatally is the high incidence of perinatal loss.

Ostium primum atrial septal defects or partial atrioventricular septal defects should always be detectable (see Chapter 5).

From experience with neonates it has been established that ventricular septal defects of greater than half the aortic root size will be of functional significance in infancy[28]. The mean aortic root size is between 2 and 4 mm at 16–20 weeks gestation (Figure 2.10). The resolution of current ultrasound equipment is between 1 and 2 mm. Thus it is only after 20 weeks gestation that defects potentially of functional importance can be confidently excluded. Our examination schedule has therefore evolved in the last six years such that the first visit at 18 weeks is to establish connections, and the second visit at 24 weeks to exclude more minor anomalies. Very small ventricular septal defects, as in postnatal life, can never be categorically excluded. Isolated small ventricular septal defects are not important if overlooked. However, it should be remembered that multiple small defects may be overlooked and these can be life-threatening. This is a further confidence limit of the technique of which the operator should be aware.

Ventricular septal defects can be seen in the perimembranous inlet, trabecular or the outlet septum as in postnatal life. A perimembranous defect with inlet extension is seen in Figure 8.3. The two atrioventricular valves and the atrial septum meet at the crux of the heart but the ventricular septum is deficient at this point. This can be distinguished from the atrioventricular septal defects illustrated in Chapter 5. Care should be taken to differentiate this defect from the appearance of dropout below the two AV valves (Figure 1.6). Dropout is seen when the beam is parallel to this thin part of the septum (positions 1 and 2 in Figure 1.5). In a ventricular septal defect a bright dot represents the end of the ventricular septum, whereas in dropout the septum fades below the valves. Imaging the four-chamber view with the beam perpendicular to this part of the septum will help to differentiate dropout from a real defect (positions 2 or 4 in Figure 1.5). When imaging with the beam perpendicular to the septum, the septum will always appear intact unless there is a real defect.

Another large inlet septal defect is shown in Figure 8.4. The right ventricle in this fetus was seen to be greater in size than the left. In other views the pulmonary artery was found to be larger than the aorta. These findings raised the suspicion of coarctation of the aorta, a fact confirmed postnatally. A further finding which could be examined on the moving image was that the tricuspid valve attachment was to the crest and left side of the ventricular septal defect. Thus there was also straddling of the tricuspid valve.

A small trabecular ventricular septal defect is seen in Figure 8.5. Sometimes such defects can be seen to open fully during diastole (Figure 8.6a) and narrow during systole (Figure 8.6b). The defect can be seen to open out just below the insertion of the moderator band into the right side of the septum.

Outlet or malalignment ventricular septal defects are typically seen in tetralogy of Fallot, truncus arteriosus or with pulmonary atresia (see Chapter 6). A malalignment ventricular septal defect may occur as an isolated defect, but this may be impossible to distinguish from tetralogy of Fallot, particularly in early pregnancy before the infundibular stenosis of tetralogy has developed and if the pulmonary artery is a normal size. The differentiation between the two conditions will not materially affect counselling the parents prenatally – both conditions will require operation with a similar surgical mortality.

Figures 8.7a and 8.7b illustrate a commonly recognized artefact. This is a densely echogenic region in the body of the left ventricle, related to the medial papillary muscle of the mitral valve. It is seen in over 1 in 50 studies, is always in the same place and of the same appearance, and is never associated with evidence of obstruction or regurgitation of the mitral valve. It is not an 'arcade' lesion which is a condition of the mitral valve in which the papillary muscles are fused together. Postnatal follow-up of patients showing this artefact, named 'golf ball in the left ventricle' as a descriptive term, has revealed no clinical signs related to the lesion. Postnatal echocardiography will show the lesion, but it is much less obvious than prenatally. This perhaps accounts for the fact that this lesion has not to our knowledge been commonly recognized postnatally. The histology of this lesion is probably fibrous tissue, but as no patient with this appearance has died this is as yet conjecture. Care should be taken to differentiate this lesion from a cardiac tumour.

Tumours are commonly multiple, may be anywhere within the cardiac mass, and produce signs of obstruction to blood flow. They will commonly increase in size during pregnancy. They have formed 4% of our cases of abnormalities detected prenatally, a much higher proportion than would be expected in a series of neonates. This can be explained by the fact that all three of our three cases of continued pregnancies resulted in intrauterine death. The histology of multiple tumours in our experience has always been rhabdomyoma, in turn indicating tuberose sclerosis[29]. Single tumours are more likely to be fibromas. Figures 8.8 to 8.11 illustrate the cases of cardiac tumour detected. The case illustrated in Figure 8.8 shows a single round lesion obstructing the mitral valve and producing non-immune hydrops fetalis. The case illustrated in Figure 8.9 shows a huge tumour in the ventricular septum obstructing both inflow and outflow of both ventricles. There were additional smaller tumours on the ventricular walls. This case again presented with fetal hydrops. The case illustrated in Figure 8.10 was examined at 18 weeks gestation when no tumour was detected. By 22 weeks gestation a tumour filled the whole right ventricular cavity. There were other tumours in the cavity of the left ventricle. By autopsy after termination of pregnancy, one week later, the largest tumour had herniated through the tricuspid valve into the right atrium. Growth of cardiac tumour has also been seen in a further case observed initially at 28 weeks gestation. Mutiple tumours could be seen in the right atrium and right ventricle and almost filling the left ventricular cavity (Figure 8.11). By 32 weeks gestation tumours had increased in size and there was evidence of obstruction to left ventricular outflow which had not been demonstrable previously. This is seen in the Doppler tracing (Figure 8.12a) showing a 2 m s^{-1} velocity of flow in the ascending aorta. The appearance of the left ventricular outflow tract at this time is seen in Figure 8.12b. It is perhaps surprising that cardiac tumours are not more commonly recorded in stillbirth autopsy series, but part of the explanation may lie in the fact that at least two of our four cases would probably have resulted in intrauterine death before 28 weeks gestation. Autopsy is not always performed in such cases.

Primary endocardial fibroelastosis is an uncommon condition in which there is hypertrophy of the left and right ventricles in association with dense endocardial thickening. Two cases have been observed both presenting in late pregnancy with fetal hydrops and both dying within hours of birth. Figure 8.13 illustrates one case: the heart was enlarged and thick-walled. The endocardial surface was densely echogenic. Both ventricles were poorly contracting with reduced flow in both great arteries. Figure 8.14 shows another case with similar appearance and presentation in which there was a laminated structure in the apex of the left ventricle 'filling in' the ventricular cavity. There was minimal flow into and out of the left ventricle and it was postulated that this could be an apical thrombus. This indeed proved to be the case at autopsy, a densely adherent 'old' thrombus being found in the apex of the left ventricle.

Secondary endocardial fibroelastosis commonly occurs in association with left-sided obstructive lesions, e.g. critical aortic stenosis or hypoplastic left heart syndrome and is confined in these cases to the left side of the heart. Such a case has been illustrated in Chapter 6. This should be distinguished from the primary form of the condition.

Figure 8.15 shows an infiltrative cardiomyopathy which may have been due to a mitochondrial myopathy. The mother presented in late pregnancy with fetal hydrops. The heart was dilated, hypertrophied and poorly contracting. The autopsy specimen was suggestive of Pompe's disease but histology suggested mitochondrial disease. The echocardiographic appearance in either disease is of an infiltrative cardiomyopathy affecting both sides of the heart.

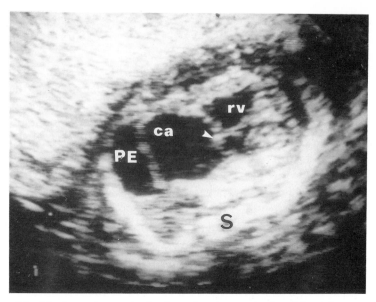

Figure 8.1 The heart is seen in the four-chamber projection. The only part of the atrial septum seen is a small stub at the insertion of the two atrioventricular valves (arrow). There is also a pericardial effusion

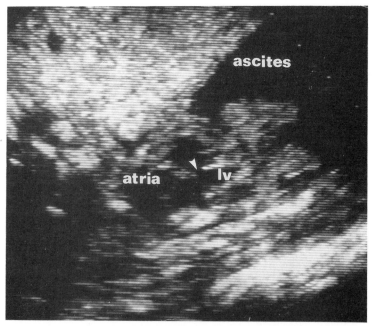

Figure 8.2 There is a small trabecular ventricular septal defect (arrow). The normal appearance of differential insertion of the two atrioventricular valves was present in this fetus, this excluding an atrioventricular septal defect

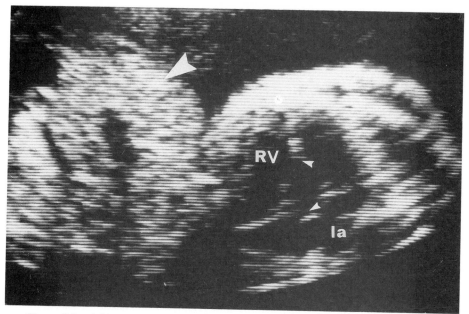

Figure 8.3 A large ventricular septal defect is seen between the two small arrows. The crest of the septum ends in a brighter dot in contrast to the common appearance of dropout in this region where the septum 'fades' below the atrioventricular valves, when the ultrasound beam is parallel to the septum. The large arrow indicates a large exomphalos which was also present in this fetus

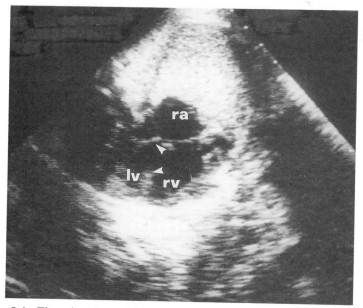

Figure 8.4 There is a large inlet septal ventricular defect seen between the two arrows. On the moving image the tricuspid valve was seen to straddle the defect. The right ventricle is dilated relative to the left due to coarctation of the aorta

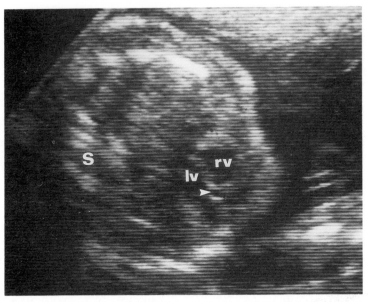

Figure 8.5 A small trabecular VSD is seen positioned just below the moderator band in the right ventricle

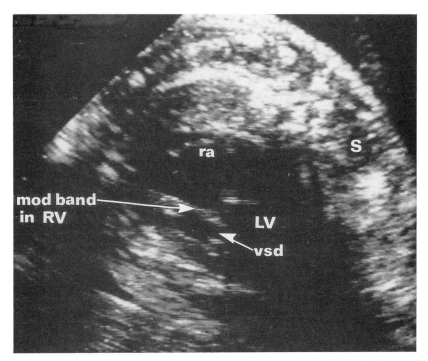

Figure 8.6a   The heart is seen in the four-chamber projection. A ventricular septal defect can be seen in diastole between left ventricle and right ventricle just below the moderator band

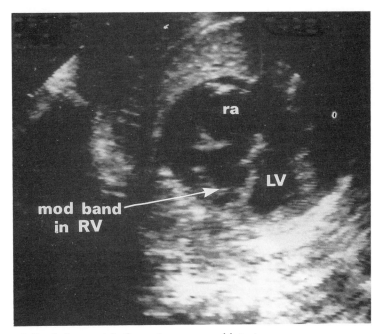

Figure 8.6b   In late systole the septum appeared intact

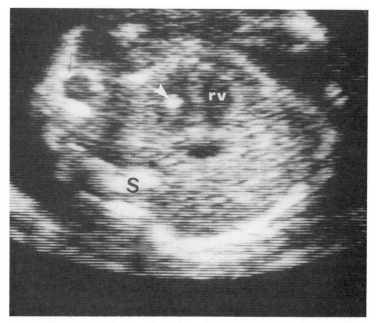

Figure 8.7a The heart is seen in a low four-chamber view. A dense echogenic mass is seen in the mid cavity of the left ventricle close to the ventricular wall (arrow). This artefact is always in the same position. There is no left atrial enlargement suggesting mitral obstruction. The mitral valve could be seen to be opening freely on the moving image

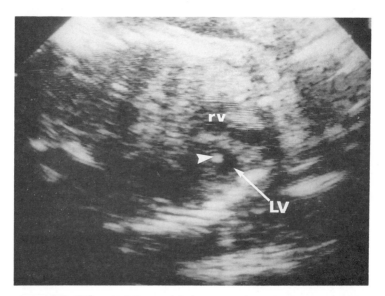

Figure 8.7b Examining the left ventricle in short axis projection shows this mass to be related to the medial papillary muscle of the mitral valve (arrow)

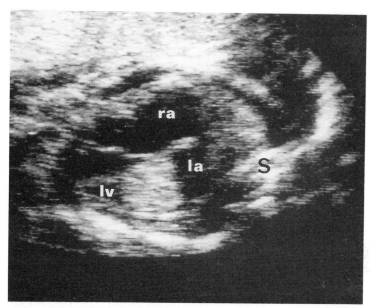

Figure 8.8   The heart is seen in the four-chamber projection. A large tumour is seen obstructing the mitral valve. The heart is dilated and there is evidence of cardiac failure

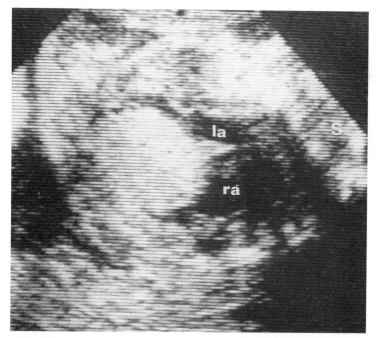

Figure 8.9   The heart is seen in the four-chamber projection but both the left and right ventricular chambers are compressed by a large tumour in the intraventricular septum

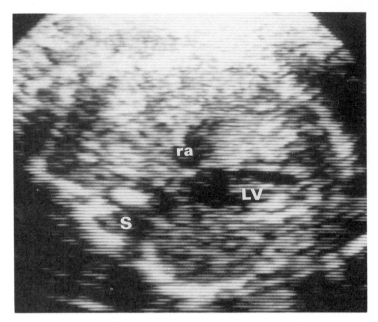

Figure 8.10   A tumour fills the right ventricular cavity, at 22 weeks gestation. Additional small tumours were seen in the cavity of the left ventricle. No discernible tumour was visible in the study performed at 18 weeks gestation

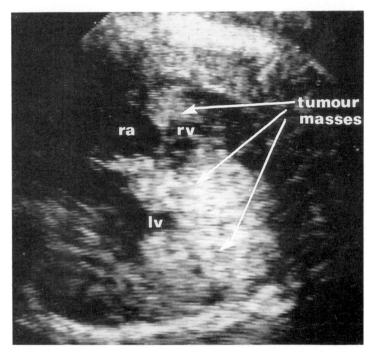

Figure 8.11   Multiple tumours are seen in this four-chamber projection. They almost completely obscure the cavity of the left ventricle

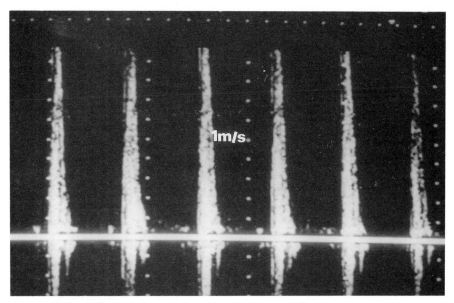

Figure 8.12a   The Doppler sample volume in the ascending aorta detected a velocity of $2\,m\,s^{-1}$, about twice the expected value (see Chapter 3). Examination of aortic velocity had been in the normal range four weeks previously

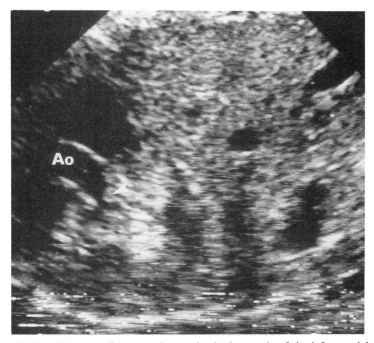

Figure 8.12b   The ascending aorta is seen in the long axis of the left ventricle. The ventricular cavity is obscured by tumour tissue. There is a tumour (arrow) encroaching on the left ventricular outflow tract. This tumour had enlarged and become obstructive between the 28 and 32 week scans

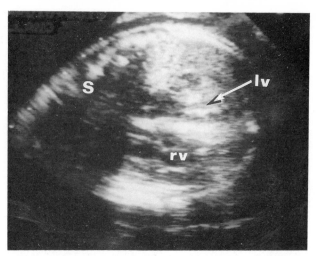

Figure 8.13 The heart was dilated and poorly contracting. The ventricular walls could be seen to be hypertrophied and densely echogenic

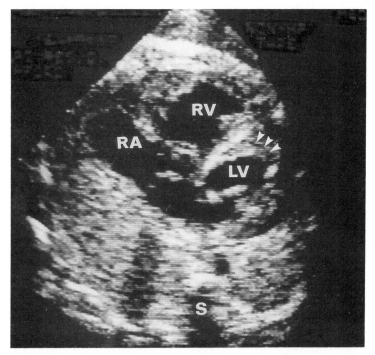

Figure 8.14 The heart was dilated and poorly contracting. There was a lamellated mass in the apex of the left ventricle (arrows) which could be differentiated from the ventricular wall because of a difference in tissue characteristics. The endocardial surface of both ventricular walls appeared increased in echogenicity. This was a case of severe primary endocardial fibroelastosis

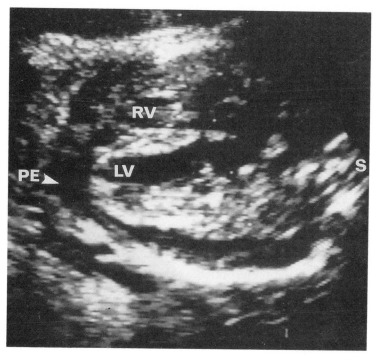

Figure 8.15   The heart is enlarged and thick-walled. It contracted poorly. There is evidence of pleural and pericardial effusion. The appearance is that of an infiltrative cardiomyopathy

CHAPTER 9

Abnormal echocardiographic appearances secondary to extracardiac lesions

There are some extracardiac anomalies which can produce a secondary effect on the heart. This can lead to an abnormal echocardiogram which can be wrongly interpreted.

HYPERTROPHIC OBSTRUCTIVE CARDIOMYOPATHY OF RENAL DISEASE

We have observed, in various forms of severe renal disease, the heart to be abnormally thick-walled with septal hypertrophy and ventricular free wall hypertrophy (Figure 9.1). The cavities of both chambers are obliterated during systole. There is evidence of obstruction to outflow i.e. mid-diastolic closure of the aortic valve and increased velocity over the left ventricular outflow tract. There is often systolic anterior motion of the mitral valve. This appearance of a hypertrophic cardiomyopathy is only seen with severe oligohydramnios in our experience. The renal pathology occurring in association can be renal agenesis, obstructive uropathy or polycystic disease. Evidence in fetal animals subjected to nephrectomy suggests they develop hypertension[30]. We assume that this fetal cardiac appearance may be secondary to severe hypertension. A similar echocardiographic appearance has been described in children with renal disease. It is not known how the associated cardiac disease affects fetal outcome, as all the pregnancies in which this was seen presented in the midtrimester. The pregnancy was terminated in four cases and intrauterine death occurred in one.

DIAPHRAGMATIC HERNIA

A left-sided diaphragmatic hernia will distort the cardiac position making evaluation of the heart difficult. As has been discussed earlier, displacement of the major blood vessels in the abdomen can confuse the normal identification of atrial situs. The orientation and relation of arterial vessels in the upper thorax can also be difficult to analyse. However, we have observed a more direct effect on the heart, that of left ventricular compression. The two ventricles appear disproportionate, with left ventricular size being well below that expected for gestational age. Careful examination shows a patent mitral and aortic valve although the left ventricular size may be in the hypoplastic left heart range. Figures 9.2a and 9.2b illustrate two such cases. The literature suggests that left ventricular hypoplasia is a real finding in autopsy specimens and that this is a major cause of the high rate of neonatal loss in this condition[31]. However, early operation in our cases allowed us to observe left ventricular size increasing into the normal range by three months of age. The infants remain alive and well with normal echocardiograms. It is important that this appearance is not incorrectly interpreted as primary cardiac anomaly. Although it may indicate severe mediastinal displacement and lung compression, therefore suggesting a poor prognosis, it does not necessarily imply a fatal outcome.

PLEURAL EFFUSIONS

These can be due to many different causes including cardiac failure and lymphatic obstruction at the thoracic inlet from a variety of causes. They can occur in association with chromosomal anomalies. Sometimes no aetiology can be found. Occasionally a small unilateral effusion can be intermittent and of no significance. The pleural effusion of cardiac failure tends to be relatively small. Gross pleural effusions can occur and tend not to have a cardiac aetiology (Figure 9.3). The distortion of the cardiac connections above and below the heart can make the interpretation of venous and arterial connections difficult. Cardiac compression can produce a false impression of left ventricular hypoplasia in the same way as a diaphragmatic hernia (Figure 9.4). It is not known why the left ventricle should be preferentially compressed compared to the right. Although in fetal life the left ventricle in this case was less than half the normal size for gestation and less than half the right ventricular size, autopsy one week later showed two ventricles of similar size. It is postulated that increased intrapleural pressure was producing this misleading appearance in life.

PERICARDIAL EFFUSIONS

It has been stated that a pericardial effusion is an early sign of intrauterine cardiac failure[32]. This is not so. It is common to see a thin line of pericardial fluid when the ultrasound beam is perpendicular to the ventricular wall and pericardial surface. This is perfectly normal and reflects the high degree of resolution of the ultrasound beam in this direction (Figure 9.5). Small pericardial effusions are common in intrauterine cardiac failure due to structural heart disease or arrhythmias, but are always seen in association with gross ascites, skin oedema and usually small pleural effusions.

Where intrauterine cardiac failure is anaemic in origin there tends to be a disproportionately large pericardial effusion with the heart 'swinging' abnormally within the pericardial sac (Figure 9.6). Anaemia is most commonly due to immune disease, but there are many other causes of fetal anaemia. The fetal heart is dilated, the right more than the left. There is increased blood flow velocity through the cardiac valves particularly on the right side of the heart. A fetal blood sample in such a case is an important part of the diagnostic work-up.

A condition of special note where anaemia occurs is that of twin–twin transfusion. This occurs only in monovular twins where one twin becomes anaemic in favour of the other becoming polycythaemic. The anaemic twin becomes smaller than the other and develops fetal hydrops. This twin is then in danger of intrauterine death and this is an indication for delivery if the fetuses are sufficiently mature. Eventually both twins becomes hydropic and the rate of fetal loss in this situation is high.

DIABETES MELLITUS

The macrosomic baby of a diabetic mother is frequently found on echocardiography in postnatal life to have a transient hypertrophic cardiomyopathy. Although we have not observed this appearance prenatally it seems likely that this can occur prior to delivery. In the postnatal form the free walls of both ventricles and particularly the ventricular septum are hypertrophied[33]. Signs of mild obstruction to outflow from the right or left ventricles are common. Such an appearance should be easy to recognise as the transient form of cardiac hypertrophy in the fetus of a diabetic mother. It does not appear to occur in the absence of macrosomia which will be evident from many ultrasonic parameters.

EXTRACARDIAC ANOMALIES COMMONLY ASSOCIATED WITH STRUCTURAL CONGENITAL HEART DISEASE

It is important to examine the heart in every case of fetal anomaly detected by ultrasound. However, some anomalies are more closely associated with heart disease than others. Exomphalos will be asociated with heart disease in nearly a third of cases, an example being seen in Figure 9.7. The most commonly associated cardiac lesions will be tetralogy of Fallot, or ventricular septal defect. The combination of heart disease and exomphalos will strongly suggest chromosome anomaly, trisomies 18 or 21. Even with normal chromosomes cardiac disease will adversely influence the prognosis for the surgical correction of exomphalos in the neonate. Duodenal atresia will be associated in at least a third of cases with an atrioventricular septal defect, with trisomy 21 as the underlying cause. Cystic hygroma will be due to Turner's syndrome in about half the cases. A careful search in this condition should be made for evidence of aortic arch anomalies, particularly coarctation (see Chapter 7). A diaphragmatic hernia occurring in association with structural heart disease will again raise the suspicion of trisomy 21. Figure 9.8 shows a left-sided diaphragmatic hernia behind the heart. There is in addition a complete atrioventricular septal defect. Occasionally rocker bottom feet, or cleft lip and palate (Figure 9.9) are identified on ultrasound. Such anomalies are frequently associated with chromosome trisomies. A ventricular septal defect is almost invariably an additional finding if the heart is examined.

FETAL HYDROPS

This may be due to many causes. However, there will be either structural heart disease or an arrhythmia as the cause in 25% of the cases. Structural heart disease tends to be severe and complex and if intrauterine failure has already supervened, the prognosis is poor, intrauterine death being a common early outcome. Right ventricular dilatation may occur in association with intrauterine cardiac failure whatever the aetiology, and should be distinguished from the ventricular disproportion occurring in association with coarctation of the aorta or total anomalous pulmonary venous drainage.

Thus many extracardiac anomalies can produce abnormal echocardiographic signs which may be open to misinterpretation. There are probably many more conditions which we have not yet encountered. It is important always to consider the fetus as a whole, accurately and completely to document echocardiographic findings, and also to have the rest of the fetus carefully examined by an experienced sonographer.

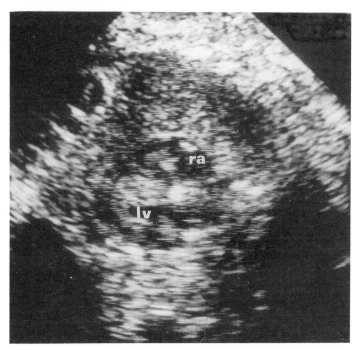

Figure 9.1 The heart is seen in the four-chamber projection. The image quality is poor due to oligohydramnios. The right and left ventricular walls are thickened. The interventricular septum is particularly hypertrophied. The cavity size of both ventricles is reduced

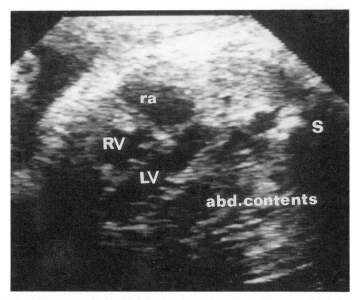

Figure 9.2a The heart is imaged in the four-chamber projection. The abdominal contents fill the left chest displacing the heart into the right chest. The left ventricle and left atrium are much smaller than the right-sided chambers. Comparison with normal growth charts indicate a fairly severe degree of left ventricular hypoplasia. However, patent mitral and aortic valves were seen with forward flow through both valves on Doppler examination

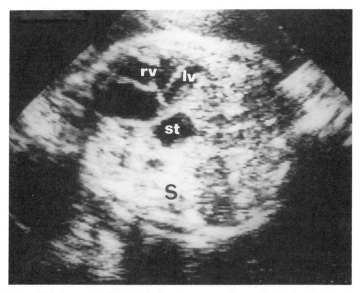

Figure 9.2b The heart is displaced, by the stomach and intestines, into the right chest. The left ventricle is conspicuously smaller than the right. This is a functional compression and should not be confused with underlying primary cardiac anomaly. This degree of 'left ventricular hypoplasia' is reversible

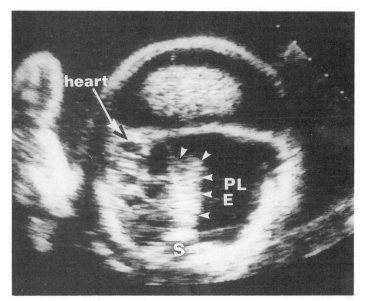

Figure 9.3 There is a large, particularly right-sided pleural effusion. The four chambers of the heart can be seen. The lung fields (arrows) are compressed by the effusion. This appearance of a gross pleural effusion, especially if unilateral, is not suggestive of cardiac failure

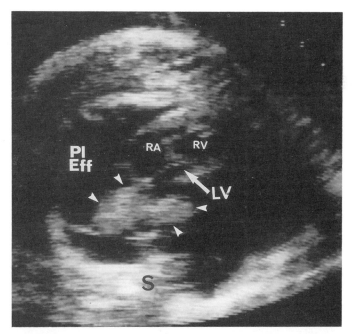

Figure 9.4 The heart is seen in the four-chamber view. There are large pleural effusions. The lungs are compressed (arrows) within the fluid. The left ventricle is minute in comparison to the right ventricle. At autopsy the two ventricles were not as strikingly different in size. It is suggested that the tension of pleural fluid was compressing the left ventricle during life, producing the appearance of primary left ventricular hypoplasia

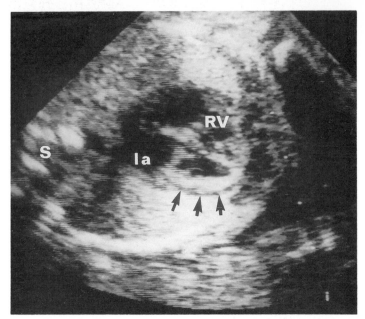

Figure 9.5 A thin rim of pericardial fluid (arrows) is seen within the pericardial sac. This is a normal appearance. It reflects the high degree of resolution of the ultrasound beam in this projection, when the myocardium can be clearly differentiated from the pericardial wall

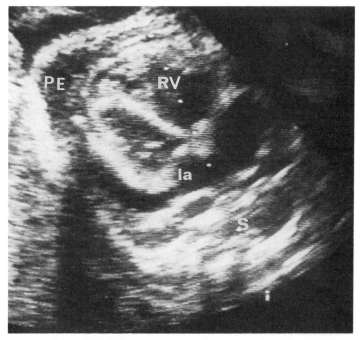

Figure 9.6 A large pericardial effusion is seen. The heart can appear unusually thick-walled but this is just because the ventricles are outlined by fluid. In the moving image the heart appears to swing abnormally with each contraction within the fluid. This appearance is commonly associated with fetal anaemia from any cause

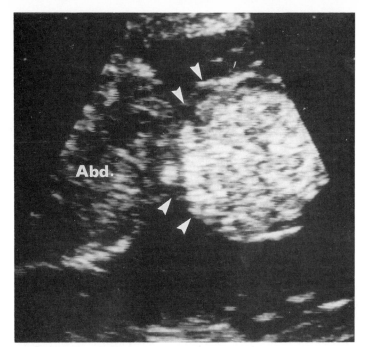

Figure 9.7 The junction of the anterior abdominal wall with an exomphalos is seen. Detection of this defect should prompt a thorough examination of the fetal heart. The majority of fetuses with congenital heart disease and exomphalos will have trisomy 18, some will have trisomy 21. A few have exomphalos, congenital heart disease and normal chromosomes. The prognosis in this situation for correction of the exomphalos will depend on the severity of the congenital heart disease

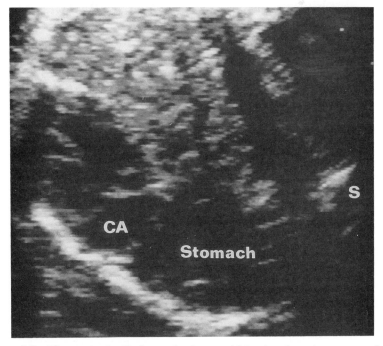

Figure 9.8 The stomach displaces the heart within the chest in a case of diaphragmatic hernia. There is a common atrium and complete atrioventricular septal defect found in the heart. This fetus had trisomy 18

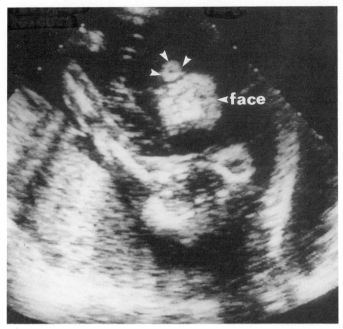

Figure 9.9 The free-floating maxillary process of a bilateral cleft palate is seen by cutting up and down through the anterior face. This occurred in association with a chromosomal trisomy

CHAPTER 10

Miscellaneous rare anomalies of cardiac structure

ECTOPIA CORDIS

This is a defect of the anterior chest wall. It can be of varying severity, from a defect of the entire chest and abdominal wall to a small defect in the lower thorax only, exposing pericardial tissue. Figure 10.1 illustrates a severe case of ectopia cordis where the whole heart was lying free in the amniotic fluid. The venous and arterial connections of the heart were elongated and distorted. There was also an intracardiac abnormality in this heart, namely tricuspid and pulmonary atresia. Intrauterine death is the most common outcome in cases of ectopia cordis, only a few surviving to delivery. Corrective operation for this defect is rarely successful.

CONJOINT TWINS

When twins are joined at the thorax there is a wide variation in the possible cardiac structures. There may be two hearts joined only by pericardial tissue, through a complete range of appearances to one heart completely shared and intermingled. Figure 10.2 shows an example of one case where the twins lay facing each other with the heart completely shared between the thoraces. There were three atria, one right and two left; and two ventricles of equal size, a right and a left with an additional rudimentary left ventricle. Two aortas arose from the main left ventricle and were distributed to each twin (Figure 10.3). There were two normally related great arteries to one twin with pulmonary atresia in the other twin. There was a large inlet ventricular septal defect (Figure 10.4).

A more recent case (Figure 10.5) has proved less easy to elucidate. There appear to be two ventricles with a ventricular septal defect, two great arteries and two atrioventricular valves. The cardiac structure is shared totally between the two thoraces. No main pulmonary artery was found in either twin although a small right pulmonary artery lay beneath each aortic arch.

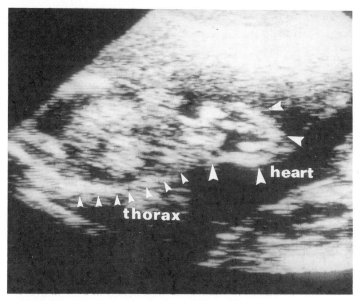

Figure 10.1 The heart is seen extruded from the fetal thorax. It lies freely in the amniotic fluid. It swung abnormally with each contraction in a similar fashion to the appearance seen with a large pericardial effusion

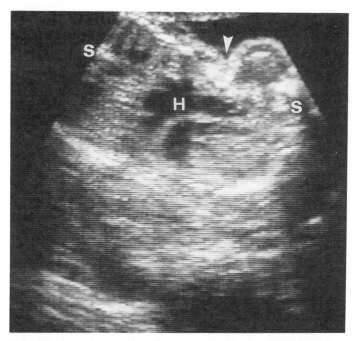

Figure 10.2 The heart is seen shared between both twins. The thoraces are joined at the arrow. The spine of the left-sided twin is just out of the picture to the left. The two twins were almost directly facing each other

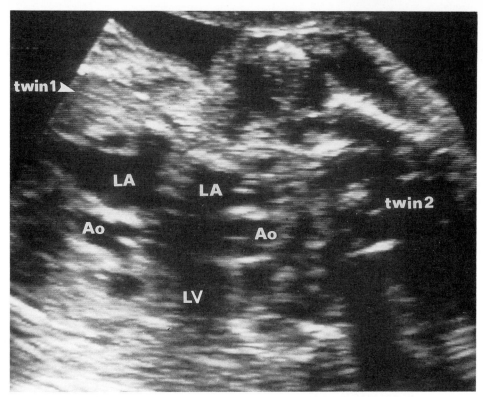

Figure 10.3 Two left atria were seen, draining to a single left ventricle via two patent mitral valves. Two aortas arose from the left ventricle to pass in opposite directions towards each twin

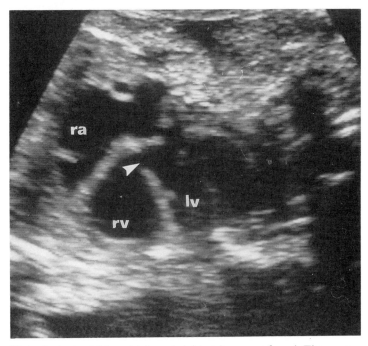

Figure 10.4 A single right ventricle and right atrium were found. There was an inlet ventricular septal defect between this and the left ventricle

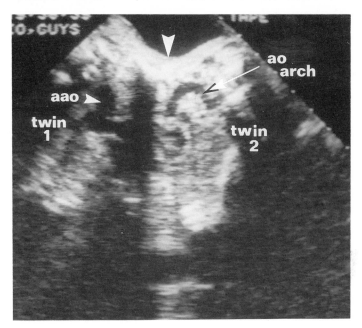

Figure 10.5 Two aortic arches were found distributed to each fetus. No main pulmonary artery could be found in either fetus. There appeared to be two ventricles. The right pulmonary artery under each arch was very small. The two thoraces joined at the arrow

CHAPTER 11

Arrhythmias

The normal fetal heart rate is around 140 beats per minute falling slightly towards term to around 130 beats per minute. Short episodes of sinus bradycardia, lasting several seconds, are common in early pregnancy and are of no pathological significance. Sinus tachycardia of up to 180–190 beats per minute are common particularly in late pregnancy and tend to be associated with fetal movement. However, a bradycardia of less than 100 beats per minute sustained for more than a few minutes, tachycardia of over 220 per minute, or frequent dropped beats (defined as more than 1 in 10) constitute arrhythmias. Such arrhythmias must be investigated by echocardiography.

The echocardiographic investigation of an arrhythmia involves examination of cardiac structure, looking for evidence of cardiac failure and M-mode echocardiographic evaluation of the rhythm disturbance. The examination of cardiac structure has already been described. Cardiac failure is evidenced by right ventricular dilatation, fetal ascites, skin oedema, and pleural or pericardial effusion. Abdominal fluid is usually the first and most readily detectable site of fluid collection. The M-mode echocardiographic evaluation of an arrhythmia involves the simultaneous recording of atrial and ventricular contraction. This is best achieved by imaging the aortic root in short axis and positioning the M-line through the aorta and left atrium (Figure 2.8). Ventricular contraction can then be inferred from the opening of the aortic valve and atrial contraction can be seen directly. In the normal heart every ventricular contraction is preceded by atrial contraction with a fixed time relationship of less than 100 ms (Figure 11.1).

BRADYCARDIAS

There are three possible causes for a sustained fetal heart rate below 100 beats per minute: profound fetal distress; blocked atrial ectopic beats; complete heart block.

Profound fetal distress

Not infrequently a slow heart rate is noted in a hydropic fetus. Fetal movement is diminished. Doppler evaluation may show absent diastolic flow in the umbilical artery and decreased cardiac output. This combination of signs suggests imminent intrauterine death.

Blocked atrial ectopic beats

Occasionally a slow rhythm can be produced by atrial ectopic beats occurring too close to the sinus beat to transmit every beat. This can be seen on the M-mode echocardiogram (Figure 11.2). Only every second atrial contraction produces ventricular systole. This is a benign arrhythmia and for that reason it is important to distinguish it from other forms of bradycardia, which will have different prognoses.

Complete heart block

Complete heart block is diagnosed when the M-mode echocardiogram reveals a regular atrial rhythm around 140 beats per minute, with the ventricular rhythm anywhere in the range 50–100 beats per minute but totally dissociated from atrial contraction (Figure 11.3).

Isolated complete heart block

This is when the M-mode criteria described above are satisfied, in the context of a structurally normal heart. In our experience this is always associated with serological evidence of connective tissue disease. The most commonly associated antibody is anti-RO[34]. Serological evidence of connective tissue disease may predate clinical disease by many years. The pathology of complete heart block in this setting appears to be antibody-mediated fibrosis of the conducting tissue in the developing fetal heart[35]. It is important to look for connective tissue antibodies as complete heart block may (though not always) recur in subsequent pregnancies.

This form of complete heart block should have a good prognosis with careful antenatal management. The management of labour can be complicated by the fact that the cardiotocograph cannot be used as an indicator of fetal wellbeing but this should not present a serious problem to the obstetrician.

Rarely fetal hydrops develops. This would be an indication for delivery. The prognosis in this situation would depend on fetal maturity. Transabdominal pacing via chest wall puncture has been attempted in such a case, where delivery was contraindicated due to prematurity[36]. To date this has not produced a live baby although it is technically feasible. It is difficult to envisage this technique as suitable for more than short-term management as it is unlikely that a pacing wire would stay in place for long. Human fetuses are notoriously adept at pulling out intracranial or intra-abdominal drains. Also a hydropic sick fetus will lie very still but once it has recovered a little and starts moving such a wire would be liable to displacement. A pacing wire passed up through the umbilical vein may be more likely to stay in place. Either way, short-term pacing to gain an extra couple of weeks of fetal growth or to induce recovery from hydrops before delivering a premature infant may make the difference between life and death in the individual fetus. This should therefore be considered in this uncommon situation.

Complete heart block with structural heart disease

It is important to differentiate this from isolated complete heart block as the prognosis here is poor. Fetal hydrops will commonly occur and intrauterine death is a frequent outcome. Of twelve cases in our series there were four intrauterine deaths, two neonatal deaths and five pregnancies were terminated. One case which was not hydropic prenatally survives at 4/12 with complex congenital heart disease. In all twelve cases there was an atrioventricular septal defect and left atrial isomerism. Many had additional anomalies of arterial connection.

TACHYCARDIAS

Diagnosis

A tachycardia demands investigation if a rate of over 220 beats per minute is reliably recorded. Even if this arrhythmia is intermittent it should be evaluated. It is not known how quickly a fetus will develop cardiac failure if a tachyarrhythmia becomes sustained but it may be only a few days. These patients usually present between 28 weeks gestation and term, the majority around 32 weeks. Half of our 14 cases have presented in severe cardiac failure. The rhythm disturbance is evaluated by comparing atrial and ventricular contraction as before. A supraventricular tachycardia will be of sudden onset with 1-to-1 conduction, with a fixed time interval between each atrial and ventricular beat (Figure 11.4). Atrial flutter is the most common intrauterine arrhythmia in our experience. Figure 11.5 illustrates the echocardiogram in atrial flutter: the atrial wall can be seen in contract at 480 beats per minute with 2:1 block between atria and ventricles. Ventricular arrhythmias have been reported prenatally[37] although we have not yet seen an example. It should be possible to differentiate from an atrial arrhythmia by seeing a slower atrial than ventricular rate, unless there is retrograde conduction of every beat. One is often presented with a hydropic fetus in sinus rhythm where the aetiology of the hydrops could be an intermittent tachyarrhythmia. If the hydrops consist of gross ascites and skin oedema with small pericardial and pleural effusions, and some cardiac dilatation, especially if there is a history of a fast rhythm recorded at the referring hospital, long-term monitoring of heart rate should take place. Forms of fetal hydrops which do not fit the above description are unlikely to be due to arrhythmias. Treatment for an arrhythmia should not be started empirically. The rhythm disturbance must be documented echocardiographically first. This is because the therapy for an atrial tachycardia is quite different from that required for a ventricular tachycardia.

Monitoring

One of the most difficult aspects of management in fetal arrhythmias is monitoring. The cardiotocograph will go off scale above 200 beats per minute or will automatically halve the heart rate at fast rhythms. It should not be used in monitoring fetal arrhythmias. Listening to the heart rate directly or echocardiographic study are more reliable indicators but neither are suitable as long-term monitors. We have used phonocardiography for this purpose[38]. This gives a 4–8 h evaluation of heart rate. A prolonged recording is essential for management, especially in intermittent arrhythmias, and in the manipulation of fetal therapy.

Treatment

There are several treatment options – no therapy, delivery, maternal therapy, direct fetal therapy, direct current cardioversion, and transabdominal pacing.

No therapy

If there is no evidence of cardiac failure and the rhythm disturbance is intermittent, occurring for less than about 20% of an 8 h period, it is reasonable to observe the patient without treatment. Should the rhythm become sustained or hydrops develop, we feel that treatment is indicated.

Delivery

If the fetus is over 35 weeks gestation there is a case for premature delivery. If there is no hydrops, we would prefer to watch closely and deliver at the first sign of decompensation, especially if the rhythm is intermittent. It is tempting to deliver a hydropic fetus of over 35 weeks gestation in order to gain control of an arrhythmia but we have experienced a death in this group. Delivery of a hydropic fetus of less than 35/52 is unlikely to produce a successful outcome.

Maternal therapy

In our view at the present time this is the method of choice in both the non-hydropic and hydropic fetus. In atrial arrthymias, in the non-hydropic fetus, the drug of choice is digoxin. Placental transfer should be as high as 100% in this situation, therefore adequate maternal serum levels should indicate adequate fetal serum levels. If after a full week of adequate maternal levels there is no effect on fetal heart rate, it is our practice to add verapamil orally. Placental transfer of this drug is good in our experience but often large doses are necessary to achieve adequate blood levels in the mother. Several of our cases have converted to sinus rhythm prior to delivery on this treatment regime.

In the hydropic fetus the situation is much more of an emergency. In atrial tachycardias our treatment of choice at present in this situation is 10–20 mg of intravenous verapamil given to the mother over 30–60 min, monitoring continuously by echocardiography during this time. A decrease in the fetal heart rate during the injection indicates a positive response, the injection is stopped and the patient is started on oral verapamil. Sometimes digoxin is required in addition for rate control. Placental transfer remains good for verapamil in the hydropic fetus but is around 50–60% for digoxin in this situation. At least 2–3 weeks of adequate blood levels of both drugs are necessary before this combination should be considered a failure. Even after conversion to sinus rhythm, hydrops can take days or weeks to clear.

If this form of therapy does fail other maternal drugs can be

considered. Propranalol, procainamide, quinidine, flecamide and amiodarone are all possibilities. We have as yet no experience of any of
these although success has been documented with procainamide and
quinidine[39,40]. Amiodarone is poorly transmitted across the placenta[41]
and is unattractive because of its property of interference with iodine
metabolism and therefore thyroid function. Lignocaine or flecanide
are possible drugs for maternal therapy in a ventricular arrhythmia.

Direct fetal therapy

This is an option that should be considered although we have so far
not been successful with this route. It is technically possible to take a
fetal blood sample from the umbilical cord and to administer drugs
via this route[42]. It should be noted that a hydropic fetus is severely
hypoxic if blood gases are measured at this time. This point should
be remembered when deciding on any form of treatment. Ideally the
hydropic fetus should be treated to recover as quickly as possible. It
may be that to date we have not been sufficiently aggressive and that
we are producing long-term deficits. However, at the present time we
have reserved direct fetal therapy for maternal drug failure, with
evidence of worsening fetal condition. Intravenous digoxin or verapamil to the fetus, cautiously and slowly given, are both possibilities.

Direct current cardioversion

This is an attractive proposition to gain fast conversion of an arrhythmia. We are unaware of its use to date and have not used it ourselves
so far. This is because of theoretical fears of inducing premature
delivery or placental abruption. Also the mother would require to be
anaesthetized for the procedure. It is a technique which deserves
consideration and perhaps evaluation.

Transabdominal pacing

It should be possible to pace the heart by direct ventricular puncture
or peferably by threading a pacing wire into the umbilical vein and
advancing it from there into the atria or ventricles. Pacing wires from
either approach would be liable to displacement on fetal movement,
but the methods appear technically possible. We feel that pacing is
perhaps an option to be considered in the future.

Set out below for the management of arrhythmias in general and
tachycardias are our provisional flow diagrams. These are based on
our current experience but by no means form a rigid plan. During

the management of any method of fetal therapy indications of fetal wellbeing should be continually monitored – fetal growth, pulsatility index in the umbilical artery, cardiac output and degree of hydrops. Information from these indicators should be included in decision making. Diagnosis and monitoring of arrhythmias can prove difficult and both techniques require improvement. The ideal form and route of therapy is still not established.

IRREGULAR RHYTHMS

Ectopic beats, both atrial and ventricular in origin, are commonly recorded in the fetus. These can be frequent, more than 1 in 10 sinus beats. They are common in the last 10 weeks of pregnancy. Figure 11.6 illustrates a case where both atrial and ventricular premature contractions are recorded. An irregular rhythm is rarely associated with structural heart disease but it is important to exclude the possibility. Cardiac tumour, cardiomyopathy or Ebstein's anomaly are the most likely anomalies to be associated with an ectopic focus. In the context of a structurally normal heart, ectopic beats are of no pathological significance in our experience. Some workers have suggested that an irregular rhythm precedes a tachyarrhythmia but this has not been the consequence in our series of nearly 100 cases. Usually the irregular rhythm disappears spontaneously towards term or soon after birth.

A summary of our current management of arrhythmias and tachycardias is seen opposite.

CURRENT SCHEDULE FOR MANAGEMENT OF ARRHYTHMIAS

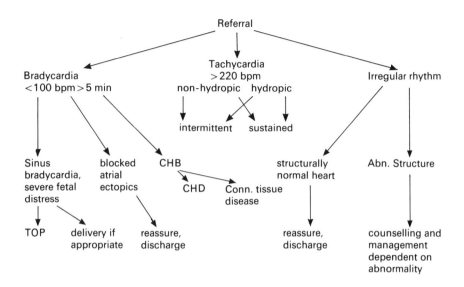

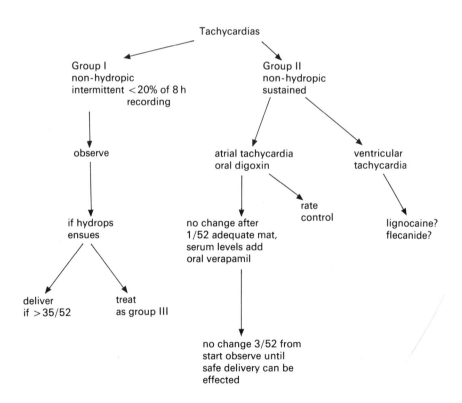

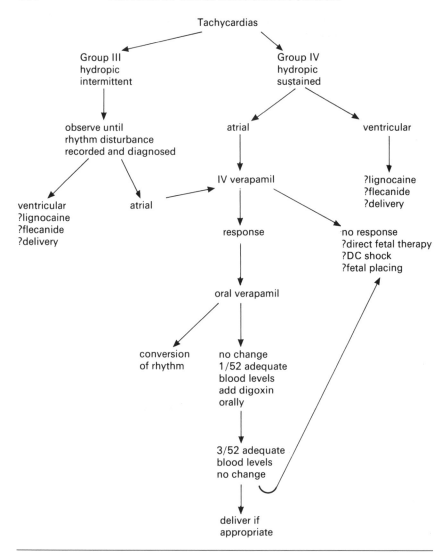

Figure 11.1 The M-line is positioned through the aorta and left atrium. Ventricular contraction can be inferred from aortic valve opening (small arrows), atrial contraction can be seen directly (larger arrows). Every ventricular contraction is preceded by an atrial contraction (analagous to the QRS complex of the ECG being preceded by a p wave). There is a constant time interval between atrial and ventricular contraction of less than 100 ms

Figure 11.2 The M-mode echocardiogram records atrial and ventricular contraction. Each ventricular contraction is preceded by an atrial contraction but the ventricular rate is only 80 beats per minute. This is because there are premature atrial contractions occurring, close to the sinus atrial contraction. The ectopic focus produces an atrial contraction but does not produce a ventricular response because the ventricle is still refractory when this stimulus occurs

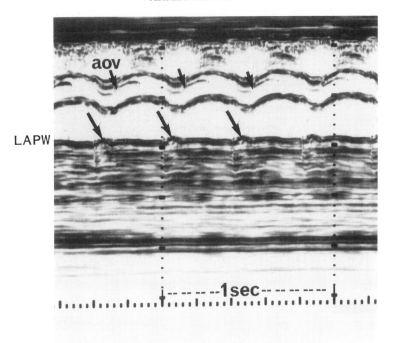

Figure 11.1

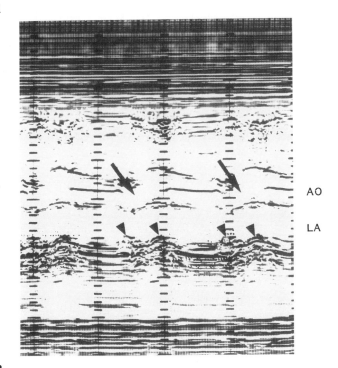

Figure 11.2

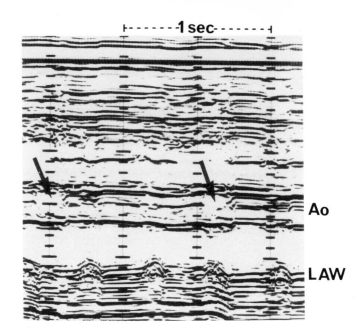

Figure 11.3

Supraventricular Tachycardia

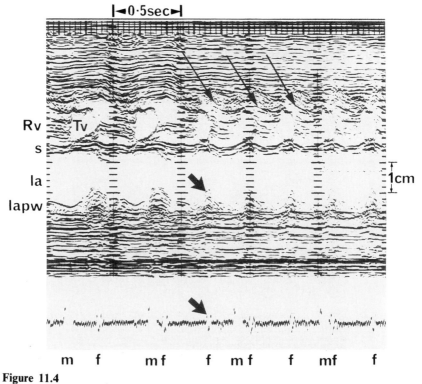

Figure 11.4

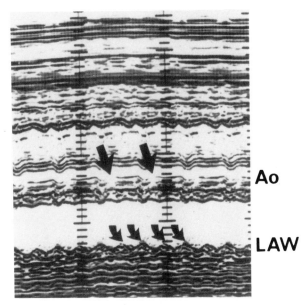

Figure 11.5 The aorta and left atrium are recorded by M-mode. The atrial wall is seen to contract at 480 beats per minute (smaller arrows) with a ventricular response to every second contraction (larger arrows). This then is atrial flutter with 2 to 1 block

Figure 11.3 The M-mode echocardiogram records the aorta and left atrium. Ventricular contraction is occurring at approximately 60 beats per minute (arrows). Atrial contraction is seen to be at a rate of about 140 beats per minute and completely dissociated from ventricular contraction. This, therefore, is complete heart block

Figure 11.4 The M-line is positioned through the right ventricular wall and left atrium. The fast rhythm shows a sudden onset (small arrows) which is against this being a sinus tachycardia. Also against this being a sinus tachycardia is the rate, which is 220 beats per minute. Ventricular contraction starts at the point indicated by the longer arrows. This has a fixed and constant relationship with each atrial contraction

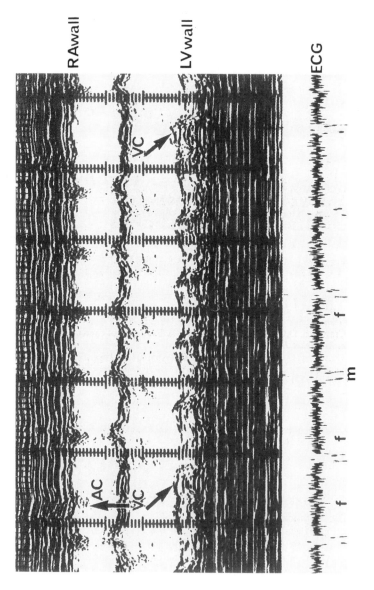

Figure 11.6 The M-mode beam crosses the right atrial and left ventricular walls. A premature atrial contraction can be seen to occur (AC) on this tracing. Also two premature ventricular contractions are seen (VC)

References

1. Allan, L.D., Tynan, M.J., Campbell, S., Wilkinson, J. and Anderson, R.H. (1980). Echocardiographic and anatomical correlates in the fetus. *Br. Heart J.,* **44,** 444–451
2. Allan, L.D., Little, D., Campbell, S. and Whitehead, M. (1981). Fetal ascites associated with congenital heart disease. *Br. J. Obstet. Gynaecol.,* **88,** 453–455
3. Allan, L.D., Tynan, M.J., Campbell, S. and Anderson, R.H. (1981). Normal fetal cardiac anatomy – a basis for the echocardiographic detection of abnormalities. *Prenatal Diag.,* **1,** 131–139
4. Allan, L.D., Tynan, M.J., Campbell, S. and Anderson, R.H. (1981). Identification of cardiac malformations by echocardiography in the midtrimester fetus. *Br. Heart J.,* **46,** 358–362
5. Allan, L.D., Joseph, M.D., Boyd, E.G.C.A., Campbell, S. and Tynan, M.J. (1982). M-mode echocardiography in the developing human fetus. *Br. Heart J.,* **47,** (Suppl.), 6, 573–584
6. Allan, L.D., Anderson, R.H., Sullivan, I.D., Campbell, S., Holt, D.W. and Tynan, M.J. (1983). The evaluation of fetal arrhythmias by echocardiography. *Br. Heart J.,* **50,** 240–245
7. Allan, L.D., Crawford, D.C. and Tynan, M.J. (1984). Evolution of coarctation of the aorta in intrauterine life. *Br. Heart J.,* **52,** 471–473
8. Allan, L.D., Crawford, D.C., Anderson, R.H. and Tynan M.J. (1984). Echocardiographic and anatomical correlations in fetal congenital heart disease. *Br. Heart J.,* **52,** 542–548
9. Allan, L.D., Crawford, D.C., Anderson, R.H., Tynan, M.J. (1984). Evaluation and treatment of fetal arrhythmias. *Clin. Cardiol.,* **7,** 467–473
10. Allan, L.D. (1984). Cardiac ultrasound of the fetus. *Arch. Dis. Child.,* **59,** (Suppl.), 7, 603–604
11. Allan, L.D. (1985). Fetal cardiac ultrasound. *The Principles and Practice of Ultrasonography, in Obstetrics and Gynecology,* **15,** 211–217
12. Allan, L.D. (1985). A review of fetal echocardiography. *Echocardiography,* **4,** 1–26
13. Allan, L.D., Crawford, D.C., Anderson, R.H. and Tynan, M.J. (1985). Spectrum of congenital heart disease detected echocardiographically in prenatal life. *Br. Heart J.,* **54,** 523–526
14. Crawford, D.C., Chapman, M.G., Allan, L.D. (1985). Evaluation of fetal bradycardia. *Br. J. Obstet. Gynaecol.,* **92,** 941–944
15. Crawford, D.C., Chapman, M.G. Allan, L.D. (1985). Echocardiography in the investigation of anterior abdominal wall defects in the fetus. *Br. J. Obstet. Gynaecol.,* **92,** 1034–1036
16. Allan, L.D. (1985). Fetal echocardiography: confidence limits and accuracy. *Pediatr. Cardiol.,* **6,** 145–146
17. Allan, L.D., Crawford, D.C., Sheridan, R. and Chapman, M.G. (1986). Aetiology of non-immune hydrops: the value of echocardiography. *Br. J. Obstet. Gynaecol.,* **93,** 223–225
18. Allan, L.D., Crawford, D.C. and Tynan, M.J. (1986). Pulmonary atresia in prenatal life. *J. Am. Coll. Cardiol.* (In press)
19. Allan, L.D., Crawford, D.C., Chita, S.K., Anderson, R.H. and Tynan, M.J. (1986). The familial recurrence of congenital heart disease in a prospective series of mothers referred for fetal echocardiography. *Am. J. Cardiol.* (In press)

20.   Allan, L.D., Crawford, D.C., Chita, S.K. and Tynan, M.J. (1986). Prenatal screening for congenital heart disease. *Br. Med. J.,* **292,** 1717–1719

21.   Rudolph, A.M. (1974). The Fetal Circulation. In: *Congenital Diseases of the Heart.* (Chicago: Year Book Medical Publishers)

22.   Kleinmann, C.S., Hobbins, J.C., Jaffe, C.C., Lynch, D.C. and Talner, N.S. (1980). Echocardiographic studies of the human fetus: prenatal diagnosis of congenital heart disease and cardiac dysrhythmias. *Pediatrics,* **65,** 1059

23.   Lewis, J.F., Kuo, L.C., Nelson, J.G., Limacher, M.C. and Quinones, M.A. (1984). Pulsed Doppler echocardiographic determination of stroke volume and cardiac output: clinical validation of two new methods using the apical window. *Circulation,* **70,** 425

24.   Meijboom, E.J., Horowitz, S., Valdes-Cruz, L.M., Sahn, D.J., Larson, D.F. and Lima, C.O. (1985). A Doppler echocardiographic method for calculating volume flow across the tricuspid valve: correlative laboratory and clinical studies. *Circulation,* **71,** 551

25.   Trudinger, B.J., Giles, W.B. and Cook, C.M. (1985). Flow velocity waveforms in the maternal neuroplacental and fetal umbilical placental circulations. *Am. J. Obstet. Gynaecol.,* **152,** 155–163

26.   Trudinger, B.J. and Cook, C.M. (1985). Umbilical and uterine artery fow velocity waveforms in pregnancy associated with major fetal abnormality. *Br. J. Obstet. Gynaecol.,* **92,** 666–670

27.   Rose, V., Gold, R.J.M., Lindsey, G. and Allen, M. (1985). A possible increase in the incidence of congenital heart defects among the offspring of affected parents. *J. Am. Coll. Cardiol.,* **6,** 376–382

28.   Canale, T.M., Saln, D.T., Allen, H.D., Goldberg, S.J., Valdes-Cruz, L.M. and Ovitt, T.W. (1981). Factors affecting real-time cross-sectional echocardiographic imaging of perimembranous ventricular septal defects. *Circulation,* **63,** (Suppl.), 3, 689.

29.   Davies, M.J. (1975). Tumours of the Heart and Pericardium. In Pomerance, A. and Davies, M.J. (eds.) *The Pathology of the Heart,* pp. 423–440. (London: Blackwell)

30.   Binder, N.D., Anderson, D.F., Potter, D.M., Thonbury, K.L. and Faber, J.J. (1982). Normal arterial blood pressure in the nephrectomized fetal lamb. *Biol. Neonate,* **42,** 50–58

31.   Siebart, J.R., Hass, J.E. and Beckwith, J.B. (1984). Left ventricular hypoplasia in congenital diaphragmatic hernia. *J. Pediatr. Surg.,* **19,** 567

32.   DeVore, G.R. Donnerstein, R.L., Kleinman, C.S., et al. (1982). Fetal echocardiography II. The diagnosis and significance of a pericardial effusion in the fetus using real-time-directed M-mode ultrasound. *Am. J. Obstet. Gynecol.,* **144,** 693–701

33.   Gutgesell, H.P., Mullins, C.E., Gillette, P.C., Speer, M., Rudolph, M.D. and McNamara, D.G. (1976). Transient hypertrophic subaortic stenosis in infants of diabetic mothers. *J. Pediatr.,* **89,** 120–125

34.   Scott, J.S., Maddison, P.J., Taylor, P.V., Esscher, E., Scott, O. and Skinner, R.P. (1983). Connective tissue disease, antibodies to ribonucleoprotein and congenital heart block. *N. Engl. J. Med.,* **390,** 209–212

35.   McCue, C.M., Mantakas, M.E., Tingelstad, J.B. and Ruddy, S. (1977). Congenital heart block in newborns of mothers with connective tissue disease. *Circulation,* **56,** 82–89

36.   Strasburger, J.F., Carpenter, R., Smith, R.T., Deter, R. and Garson, A. (1986). Fetal transthoracic pacing for advanced hydrops fetalis secondary to complete atrioventricular block. *J. Am. Coll. Cardiol.* (In press)

37.   Muller-Schmid, P. (1959). Die paroxysmale tachykardie in utero. *Geburtschilfe Frauenheilkd.,* **19,** 401

38.   Talbert, D.G., Davies, W.L., Johnson, F., Abraham, N., Colley, N. and Southall, D.P. (1986). Wide bandwidth fetal phonography using a sensor matched to the compliance of the mother's abdominal wall. *Transactions on Biomed. Eng.,* **33,** (No.2)

39.   Dumesic, D.A., Silverman, N.H., Tobias, S. *et al.* (1982). Transplacental cardioversion of fetal supraventricular tachycardia with procainamide. *N. Engl. J. Med.,* **307,** 1128

40.   Spinnato, J.A., Shaver, D.C., Flinn, G.S., Sibai, B.M., Watson, D.L. and Marin-Garcia, J. (1984). Fetal supraventricular tachycardia: *in utero* therapy with digoxin and quinidine. *J. Am. Coll. Obstet. Gynecol.,* **64,** 730–735

41.   McKenna, W.J., Harris, L., Rowland, E., Whitelaw, A., Storey, G. and Holt, D. (1983). Amiodarone therapy during pregnancy. *Am. J. Cardiol.,* **51,** (Suppl.), 7, 1231–1233

42.   Daffos, F., Forestier, F., Pavlovsky, M.C. (1984). Fetal blood sampling during the third trimester of pregnancy. *Br. J. Obstet. Gynaecol.,* **91,** 118–121.

Index